The
Accidental
Soberista

The Accidental Soberista

KATE GUNN

Gill Books

Gill Books
Hume Avenue
Park West
Dublin 12
www.gillbooks.ie

Gill Books is an imprint of M.H. Gill and Co.

978 07171 9058 4

Copy-edited by Kristin Jensen
Proofread by Caitriona Clarke
Printed by ScandBook in Lithuania

This book is typeset in 13/18pt Garamond Premiere Pro.
The paper used in this book comes from the wood pulp of
managed forests. For every tree felled, at least one tree is
planted, thereby renewing natural resources.

A CIP catalogue record for this book is available from the
British Library.

5 4 3 2 1

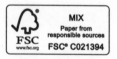

To Aodhan.
Coffee-maker, doubt-shaker.

About the author

Kate Gunn is from the seaside town of Greystones in Co. Wicklow, where she lives with her three children and her partner, Aodhan. A well-known blogger and features writer in both the UK and Irish parenting realms, Kate has written regularly for Irish newspapers and online websites. Her first book, *Untying the Knot*, was published by Orpen Press.

Contents

Introduction

There wasn't one major reason, more a few minor ones. I had an inkling that alcohol was perhaps holding me back from getting on top of my life. Plus the hangovers were getting worse. No longer just a dull headache throughout the day, at the worst times entire weekends were wiped out by one fun night I could hardly remember.

I'd also been introduced to the One Year No Beer movement by my ex-husband, who was feeling the benefits of it. So when my partner sheepishly told me he was thinking of doing 30 days alcohol free, I cautiously agreed. Our relationship was only a year old and had been built on nights out and bottles of red wine. I wondered how we would cope. Would we still entertain each other? Would I have enough to talk about without my old-time loosener friend?

I was a social drinker, usually having a few (or more) drinks two to three nights in any week. I loved red wine by the fire and cold beers in the sunshine. I couldn't possibly imagine going 'out out' and not drinking. Who could, or would, want to do that? I had been drinking pretty much since I was 16 years old – I didn't know myself or life without alcohol by my side.

Although I had been mostly alcohol free during my three pregnancies, somehow this was different. The only other time I'd done 30 days completely off alcohol was one Dry January that was so miserable I promised myself I would never, ever do it again. I even went on BBC Radio urging others not to make the same terrible mistake. 'Don't do it! Isn't January bad enough already?'

So what changed? One very simple thing: my mindset. Instead of focusing on what I was depriving myself of, I focused on what I was gaining. Such a simple but effective way of changing your life.

And now I know that the fun can mostly be had without the drink, though not that 'lost weekend' kind of fun. But then again, most of those lost weekends are actually lost from memory too, wiped out other than a few random flashes. Fun nowadays is more wholesome, more real and, weirdly, more fun.

Since being alcohol free I've been to gigs, festivals, dinners, nights out and parties – and I've had fun at all of them. Plus I've been given the added benefit of remembering them. Sure, I'm ready to head home at midnight most of the time, but I'm more than happy with that. I get to see my friends, have a good night's sleep and then I'm ready to leap out of bed the next morning, full of life and smugness. I get the best of both worlds.

Breaking free from alcohol has improved every single aspect of my life, from relationships to health to work to happiness. I feel like I have been given a wonderful gift and I want to share it with others. I want to lift the veil of alcohol so that the truth is exposed. I want you to see that giving up alcohol isn't a chore or a loss – it could be the best decision you will ever make for yourself and your life. Could it be worth trying? Would it be possible for 30 days or even a few months, just to see whether life is as good – or even much, much better – on the other side?

Chapter 1

My Drinking Career

I had gone through numerous different drinking periods in my life up to that point. Young teenage drinking, when I first experimented with vodka and orange at a friend's house party, the taste of huge shots of vodka masked by strong, sugary orange cordial. As I got drunk for the very first time, I remember being totally confused by the fact that I knew what I wanted to say but it kept coming out wrong. The vodka and orange also came out wrong at the end of the night, all over the bathroom floor. I never touched that drink again; even the scent of it would turn my stomach years later. Over the next few years I moved on to other sugar-coated drinks. Malibu and pineapple on a school exchange in France, vodka and blackcurrant in the local nightclub and, bizarrely, White Russian cocktails in my late teens. Who did I think I was, Jeff Lebowski?

In my college years, I drank whatever was cheap. Cut-price prosecco, flagons of cider, buy six get one free on Murphy's stout in the local pub with drops of sugary blackcurrant added until I learned to like the taste.

These were the days of all-day drinking sessions with my housemates, when we would stop by the local pub on our way home from a supermarket shop and fall home 12 hours later, the plastic bag of milk and BBQ beef Super Noodles long forgotten on a floor somewhere.

In my second year of university I found myself living with another girl who had the same name as me, so for that period of time we had exactly the same name and the same address. It was our party trick that we rolled out when meeting new people. One day during our first term back on campus, I got a call from the university office – could I come down and speak to them, please? Obviously, I had The Fear. Anything to do with authority when you are a living-away-from-home-revelling-in-freedom student sends nervous shivers down your spine. Were they going to kick me out? Had I done something wrong? My mind searched back to try to find what I could possibly have done that necessitated what felt like being sent to the headmaster's office. I told them I'd be straight down. The worried faces of my housemates did nothing to allay my fears.

The secretary in the office called me in. She seemed kind and smiley and I wondered if this was what a friendly assassin looked like.

'Oh, come in. Thank you for dropping over so quickly. Now, there seems to have been a bit of a mistake ...'

She explained how they had received two sets of fee payments and showed me on the printed sheet, pointing to my name and my address listed twice. 'You see? Here and here.'

I swallowed.

'So we'll just refund the second payment. We can give you a cheque if you like?'

'Um ...'

My mind raced through the possible responses: a cheque for £500 or an explanation that it was a possible mix-up. I needed to talk to my namesake.

'A cheque sounds fine,' I heard myself saying in a high-pitched squeak as she rummaged in the desk.

I ran out of the office, my face burning and my mind bursting with excitement. I still wasn't sure what to do, but I knew I had a brilliant story to tell. I raced back home to tell my housemates so that we could decide what to do. Should we tell our parents and give them the money? Or go back to the secretary to explain what we thought may have happened? Or sit on the money for a while in case they realised the error?

I fell in the door. 'You'll never guess what happened!'

It was clear to me as soon as I began to relay the events that we would not be giving that money back. We all marched straight down to the bank, cashed the cheque and went to the pub. We agreed we would spend £50 and keep the rest for a couple of months to see whether anyone came looking for it. A perfect plan. We met friends, made new friends, regaled everyone with the crazy story of what had just happened, bought drinks, tried cocktails and shared out boxes of cigarettes. We were queens in the ranks of the impoverished student lives all around us. Lottery winners, fun givers, glitter makers.

The next morning, I woke up with a sore head and a feeling of overwhelming dread coursing through my body. No, no, no, no, no. I didn't. I couldn't have. Could I? I rolled over and dragged my jeans from the floor, searching empty pockets until I found something: a £20 note wrapped around a brand new plastic lighter. It was all I had to show from the stolen money of the day before other than a few fuzzy memories of the evening.

It suddenly didn't feel like a very funny story any more. Or a perfect plan. Those first few pints had taken our carefully considered idea, crumpled it into a ball and thrown it, along with caution, to the wind. All sensible notions were pushed to one side and the only thing being carefully considered was how many drinks were in the next round I was buying.

My poor parents. They never knew their hard-earned cash had been spent on one epic student pub crawl.

My parents were moderate drinkers with more than a little love of wine. When I was a child I remember lying in bed, excited by the sounds of raucous dinner parties emanating from the room below. There were heated debates, and laughter, and sometimes songs. My father played the fiddle and would use any excuse to drag it out and show off his middling talent. I couldn't wait until I was old enough to join in.

We had a big house in a beautiful town but not much disposable income when I was growing up. One of the ways my parents decided to save money, and start a side hustle, was by going into business selling homebrew wine kits. They were already homebrew beer aficionados and we would regularly have plastic drums of beer bubbling away beside the Aga throughout the year. When it came to bottling time we were all roped in to help, sucking secret sips of golden nectar as we siphoned the beer from barrel to bottle through long clear tubes. My father was always looking for ways to perfect his latest product – a new kit, a tweaking of the recipe, better storage. This was taken to new heights the year he decided to go all natural.

I was in secondary school at the time. As the final bell of the day went and we all poured out the doors at 3:30 p.m., a strange smell hit us. What *was* that? An earthy aroma that none of us could pinpoint but all of us agreed was disgusting. As we walked towards the town, it got stronger and stronger until we were covering our faces with scarves and wrinkling our noses in disdain. We decided it must be manure – perhaps a farm truck had accidentally shed its load. I waved goodbye to my friends as we dispersed to our different houses. But the smell kept getting stronger. As I turned up the bottom of my road it hit with full force, like a big earthy shit. I practically ran up the driveway to get in my house and away from the stench. As I did I bumped into my dad, a big grin on his face.

'Want to see my hops?' he asked, clearly thrilled with himself.

Behind the hedge stood a huge mound of them. I could practically see the steam coming off them and wafting through the town. Every person I knew would soon realise that the new farm smell was coming from my home. I was aghast. I threw my school bag over my shoulder and did my best teenage strop away from him, silently screaming, 'HOW COULD YOU DO THIS TO ME?!'

As it turned out, my dad had got slightly confused with his order. He had meant to buy a small delivery to test out with his brewing, but he'd ordered 50 times what he expected so he used it for his gardening instead.

Perhaps that was why they moved on to wine. But this time, they had bigger plans. Instead of just using the homebrew to save money, they decided to make money from it too. My dad, ever the entrepreneur, had found some amazingly good wine-making kits and had decided to buy the franchise. He would sell the kits and make a profit from his sideline while kindly helping others to save on the costs of their weekend drinking.

Again, arriving from school, this time I found the kitchen overloaded with boxes of red and white wine-making kits. They stood from floor to ceiling stacked up in rows five deep. We built forts out of them and shifted in and out of our dining room chairs sideways for months. Each of the boxes displayed the face of a strange bearded man holding a glass of wine, a self-satisfied smile on his face. His eyes followed me as I poured milk on cereal and ate my Sunday roast. It's amazing that I didn't become a teetotaller at that point.

Over the weeks, the boxes didn't seem to be going anywhere. With little fanfare, my parents had decided that these kits made exceedingly good wine, so what was the point in selling them? Instead they would keep them for their own use and give some to the neighbours. For the next 10 years, those kits were rolled out – red and white wine on tap, bottles stored in kitchen cupboards. My elder sister built her teenage years on stolen bottles of it.

As teens most of us stole from our parents' drinks cabinets, making concoctions that had nothing to do with taste and everything to do with how much of each bottle we could get away with. Topping up vodka and gin bottles with a little water, leaving the precious whiskey untouched (he'd definitely notice), adding a drop of port and a splash of sherry. Usually it would all be shaken up in a jam jar to be brought to the closest field or, on really special occasions, a beach party. My lasting memory of these raids came not from a party and not from my own house, but the event will be imprinted on my mind forever more.

Myself and my best friend were at another friend's home on a Friday afternoon after school. She was supposed to be preparing the dinner for when her parents came home from work, but for reasons beyond my understanding had decided to graze on homemade cocktails instead. Ever the sensible one, I did not think this was a good idea. She continued to take a little of this and a bit of that until she was talking incoherently and I was panicked that her parents would walk in.

'She's just pretending,' my other friend said hopefully.

'Are you pretending?' I asked crossly.

She gave me a dopey smile from upside down on the bed.

'Quick, get her some coffee!' I said. I'd seen it in movies and it always worked for them.

We made it strong and black but forgot to warn her that it would be hot. She took a gulp and dropped the cup as it burned her mouth. Shit!

'Okay, water! She needs water!' We made her drink it and we poured it on her face. Unsurprisingly, it had zero impact.

'The potatooooes are in the fieeeelds,' she sang happily, presumably a reference to the unmade dinner sitting in bags on the kitchen counter.

And then the front door shut.

My friend and I froze, staring at each other with terrified eyes. Her parents.

'She hit her head!' my friend burst out as they entered the room.

Brilliant! I thought to myself. A genius explanation. Except I didn't realise that concussion shows up as confusion and can be dangerous. They hovered over her worriedly, trying to get her to look at them, but her eyes wouldn't focus. She would obviously need to see a doctor. It was Friday night, so the only option was to bundle us all in the car and drive to the nearest hospital.

The three of us sat in the backseat of their car like a teenage girl version of *Weekend at Bernie's*. We were under strict instructions not to let her go to sleep (bad for concussion, good for drunkenness). We threw panicked glances at each other, knowing that we were in deep trouble now. Should we just tell them the truth? The doctors would know instantly, of course, so we were only prolonging the agony. But neither of us could find the courage. So we sat worrying about how much trouble we would be in while her parents mistook our silence for concern over their poor daughter.

'She'll be okay, please don't worry,' they kindly consoled us while presumably wracked by their own fears. It only made things worse.

When we got to the hospital, they took her off for testing. Myself and my friend took the opportunity to inhale a couple of packets of cheese and onion crisps from a vending machine just in case there was any residual smell of alcohol on our breath. What the fuck were we going to do now? In about eight minutes they would be walking through those double doors knowing full well that their daughter was drunk, not concussed.

The doors swung open and they walked towards us.

'They want to send her for a CT scan, so we have to go to a different hospital,' they explained. I couldn't believe what I was hearing. Was this good news or bad? Were we going to get into even more trouble at the end of this or might we have just got away with it?

We said nothing and silently nodded.

Back in the car, arrive at a new hospital, out of the car, in for more tests, more waiting, more self-absorbed worrying. An hour or so later, they all walked out alongside a doctor. Time stood still.

'She's fine. No damage,' the doctor said to us. No mention of alcohol. No admonishment. Just a long, knowing stare into my eyes.

Her parents brought us McDonald's on the way home, apologising for our terrible night. We had escaped unscathed – except for the crushing guilt I felt whenever I thought about them.

Like most people at that time, my childhood was filled with grown-ups drinking for pleasure. There was no alcoholism in my own family or those around me, so drinking never seemed 'problematic' to me. It was something shiny and alluring and a little bit out of bounds. In my twenties I remember inviting my dad out for a pint with me and my friend, Eric. We sat in a local pub chatting and sharing stories, the buzz of conversation all around us and the warmth of the fire in the corner of the room. A happy glow settled on me. My dad sat smiling at me.

'What?' I asked.

'You look so content,' he said, 'like you're really at home here.'

I *was* content. I felt like a grown-up, an equal, able to hold my own in both conversation and drinking. I had come of age.

'What have we done to you?' he half joked.

I didn't know what he meant. He had to explain it to me – the drinking being normalised, the pub being a place of contentment. I scoffed at him, annoyed at how ridiculous he was being. My parents were hardly heavy drinkers. They would share a bottle of wine on a Friday and Saturday night and Dad might nurse one single precious Wild Turkey whiskey in his hand after a hard day, but a bad influence they were not. Everybody drank. I would be drinking with or without them. Stop being so foolish!

There were many blackouts during these twenty-something years. Nights I fell up the street alone and nights I fell down, turning to see if anyone had seen as I wiped the gravel from my knees. Mornings I woke up in bed not knowing how I got there, sometimes with a new friend beside me. When I think of the situations I put myself in, or my daughter doing the same, it sends a shudder of fear through me. I was very, very lucky that nothing really bad ever happened. I was not alone in these experiences or even close to the worst in my circles of friends. This was a rite of passage, the common coming of age of almost all young people in this country.

As adults we tend to cast aside those years as 'sure, everyone goes through it'. It's just part of being young, growing up and learning from our mistakes. But maybe we should all take more time to think through those experiences instead of just brushing them off. As teens we force ourselves to drink alcohol, learning to like the 'acquired' taste over time, masking what our bodies really think of it with sugar. Why do we do this? Because that's what all the people around us are doing. If everyone else is drinking, it must be fun. Adults and parents tell us not to drink while topping up their own glasses, adding to the allure of a drug we are not permitted to have.

Drinking is grown-up. It's fun. Everyone else is doing it. These are the messages our young minds are given from a very early age. How can we not buy into it?

Like many people, I have gone through periods of my life where drinking featured heavily and others where it eased off. University was full of drunken nights and all-day sessions. But after four years, a degree and a post-grad, I was ready for something different.

During my final term, a friend noticed a poster on one of the noticeboards outside the lecture hall to volunteer on behalf of the college in a range of less developed countries. I knew this was my next step in life. I arranged an interview but had absolute confidence that it was merely a formality – that place was mine.

And it was. I got a call from them to say that I was one of four selected to go to Mexico. It would be a six-week trip and they would arrange all the details.

Weeks later we travelled to Tijuana, where we would be stationed. We would be living in a Christian-run community project, which was filled with other volunteers from the likes of Mexico, Spain, Germany and America. It was like an international summer camp with Jesus. Needless to say, there was not a lot of partying going on. Not everyone was deeply religious, but everyone was there for a reason bigger than themselves. Many wanted to help the disadvantaged families that were scattered in far-reaching shanty towns all along the border, dreams of a better life halted by wire fences, guns and dogs. Others were running away from their own problems of broken relationships, overbearing parents or unexpected job losses, which suddenly seemed far less important when you saw young children picking through a rubbish dump for something that might feed their family that day.

The community became like a family to us all. Supportive, kind, sometimes argumentative, always present. We would rise early to do chores, go to prayer in the little chapel, have breakfast and then head off to our assigned towns. Mine was far up in the Mexican mountains. In those first six weeks I would take a taxi from town, squished in between old men with leather skin and cowboy hats and large, colourful women carrying woven bags and sometimes the odd live chicken. My favourite seat was the one that sat backwards in the boot of a station wagon so that I could watch the dusty road fading behind me as we wound our way up the hills.

I loved it there. Six weeks became six months and soon I was driving an old pick-up truck up to the mountains, sometimes loading kids in the back to go on little adventures with me. It was a special time. There was zero alcohol around me – its only visibility at that time was in the whispered stories of the women who had been at the harsh end of their husband's love of it the night before. My privileged, sheltered life had cracked open to reveal what was outside of it.

Towards the end of my time in Mexico, a friend came over to visit and I took two weeks off to go travelling with her. We rode trains through the Copper Canyon and horses through old colonial towns, we swam in crystal clear water and drowned ourselves in icy margaritas.

When I returned to the community, I showed one of my Mexican volunteer friends the photos. In one I sat laughing with a huge margarita glass in my hand, cheeks flushed red and a large sombrero on my head.

'*Muy feo,*' he said. Very ugly. The Mexicans are nothing if not direct.

I was annoyed and rolled my eyes. We were having FUN. It's allowed, you know? But every time I looked at the picture after that, all I saw was a fake drunken smile and unfocused eyes.

After I came home from Mexico, I entered normal life as a twenty-something-year-old. I got a job, moved out of my parents' house, got another job, moved back, earned, spent and messily navigated my way to adulthood. My good friend, Eric, was doing the same thing. He lived with his sister and brother-in-law in our hometown and we started working for the same large American computer company. One night I went over to their place for a meal out before we all hit the pub together. It was the couple's wedding anniversary, so we bought drinks, then they bought drinks, then we bought more drinks and the night continued like many others. None of which I can actually remember.

Much, much later that night we all fell home together and said our drunken goodnights. They went off to their bedroom and I got into bed beside Eric, something we would sometimes do as purely platonic friends when the convenience of staying over in each other's houses was required.

We all fell into a deep, drunken sleep.

In the early hours of the morning there was a bang and the bedroom door opened. A dark figure stood in the doorway swaying. I pretended to be asleep until it moved towards us and tried to get into bed beside me.

'Eric!' I hissed, nudging my elbow into his ribs. It took him a moment to realise what was happening, and then he was instantly on it. Ever the practical joker, he already had a plan. He moved out of the bed, allowing his brother-in-law to slide in.

'Stay there and cover your face with the duvet so that just your hair is showing. Say nothing. I'll be back in a minute.'

I still wasn't sure what was going on, but he seemed delighted with himself so I did what I was told.

Moments later, his sister burst through the door, shouting. 'Oh my God! Who the hell are you in bed with? You bastard! And on our anniversary! How could you?'

He leapt out of the bed, eyes wide with horror, double-taking between my hidden form in the bed and his furious wife.

'I … I don't know who that is. I didn't do anything!' The panic in his face was palpable. He was desperately trying to piece together the night before but couldn't find the answers in his poor, terrified, hungover brain.

'Well, let's see who it is then!' she shouted, marching over and ripping back the cover from my face.

He looked down at me with a blank, confused stare before the rest of us all fell about laughing.

'Your face!' she squealed, wiping the tears from her eyes.

Eric looked like he'd won the lottery, dancing from foot to foot at the doorway, delighting in his brilliance.

I felt bad for the poor man. He took his broken self back to bed and spent the rest of the day recovering, thoughts of 'what ifs' and 'thank Gods' racing through his mind.

I'm quite sure many, many people face that horror in life without the relief of a practical joke being at the end of it.

It wasn't long before the narrowness of living and working within a five-mile radius got to me and I began to dream of faraway places. I was 24, managing a team of technicians and compiling reports I didn't fully understand. My boyfriend at the time was an adventure-seeker and a life of spreadsheets and headsets didn't exactly set his world on fire. Instead he was planning on saying goodbye and going to Australia for a year with his wild friends. I felt safe and boring and stuck.

Australia. I'd always wanted to go. Maybe...

It wasn't long before I was cashing in my company shares, strapping on my backpack and departing on my own adventure.

After staying with friends for the first few weeks, I headed off down the coast on a free lift, visiting some weird and wonderful places along the way. Finally I arrived at a hostel in Byron Bay, just off the Gold Coast. It was pure hippieville and had been recommended to me by a dreadlocked masseuse I had met in a commune the night before. Who better to tell me where to take my life next?

I landed alone with a bag of weed in one hand, a bag of CDs in the other and an enormous backpack strapped around me like an oversized stoned tortoise.

I was given a dorm room with six others, some of whom sat outside the room on long wooden beaches, sheltered from the sun by massive palm trees. They introduced themselves and invited me out for drinks that night. They had all been staying at the hostel for weeks, having found a little piece of paradise none of them wanted to move on from. There was a group of about 10 who came from Australia, the UK, Israel, Japan and Holland who had become firm friends. I felt awkward among their obvious comradery. An outsider.

So what better way to become part of the gang than to buy rounds of drinks? I ordered shots of Irish whiskey and later that evening fell into deep and important conversations with one of them. Kristian had come to Australia from England the year before and would soon be coming to the end of his visa. We bonded over music and drinking. Kindred spirits. The future sparkled.

I woke the next day in his single dorm bed, head thumping and stomach churning. He left to get breakfast and meet the others as I spent the next eight hours vomiting, full of self-loathing. I could hear them all rehashing the fun of the night before. Someone mentioned the new girl.

'What did you *do* to her, Kristian?' one of them asked and they all laughed. I rolled over and berated my stupidity for the millionth time that day. Never again.

In the early evening, Kristian came back to check on me again and I managed to weakly rise and make my way down the path to the hostel café, where I nibbled on tiny bites of buttered toast and gingerly sipped my tea with shades on. The other diners, tanned and healthy, shot me pitying glances. I felt embarrassed and stupid.

I'm not sure if it was thanks to my sparkling personality or the big bag of weed, but it was testament to Kristian and my new friends that they didn't all dump me immediately. Fortunately, when I was well enough to speak again, they welcomed me into the fold and we all formed a special bond lasting many years in some cases and a lifetime in others.

I spent the next few years living, working or travelling between Australia, England, New Zealand and Thailand. A couple of years after first meeting, Kristian and I took three months out to explore the islands of Thailand, moving from one to another on wooden long-tail boats and living on beaches in little huts with nothing more than a hammock and a bed. It was paradise.

Our final spot before leaving to come home for Christmas was in a small rocky inlet on a small, quiet island more known as a local holiday spot for visiting Thais than for swarms of backpackers and tourists. We couldn't believe our luck finding such a perfect place to finish our trip. There was only a handful of huts at our little oasis, each nestled into rocks just above an inlet of pure, clear turquoise water. It was remote, peaceful and stunningly beautiful.

On the day of Kristian's birthday I gifted him with a Sherlock Holmes book that I had found in a second-hand store on a previous island and a bottle of precious Johnny Walker whiskey, a hard thing to find where we were. Later that night we headed out to meet some new friends at a local beach bar. We strolled through the trees as we made our way up and down the rocky headland that brought us from our hidden hideaway to the main beach.

That night we drank strong beer, local cocktails and birthday shots. We shared stories, sang songs and gave each other heartfelt compliments. We sat with the sea lapping at our ankles with twinkling fairy lights and glowing candles all around us.

And then it was time to go home. The magic had faded. We were tired and ready for bed. Kristian had had one too many celebratory drinks and was staggering uncharacteristically. I put my arm around him and manoeuvred him around the bends and up the steep inclines. At 6 foot 2 to my 5 foot 2, it wasn't an easy task. But as we got closer to home, it became harder. He wanted to stop and lie down, but I knew I couldn't let him. I cursed at him under my breath and then out loud, frustrated that he couldn't see we needed to get to the hut before he collapsed. And then, on the final hill before the path led to our inlet, he did. He lay on the path and I couldn't get him any further.

One of the workers from our place, a man who kept the grounds for the people who owned the huts, passed by below. I ran down and waved at him, pointing up the hill to where Kristian lay. We had no common language, so I made wild gestures until he followed me up the hill.

He helped me raise and walk Kristian down the hill, our arms around him as if we were all in some sort of bizarre three-legged race. And then his arm reached around a little more, until he grabbed my breast.

I leapt away, at that moment more furious than frightened.

'What are you doing?' I shouted, knowing he couldn't understand me. 'You are supposed to be helping me!' I raged.

The horror of the past hour's expedition had left me exhausted and frayed. How could he be taking advantage of the situation like this? But the problem was that I still needed him. Our hut stood just 20 metres away, but I needed him to help get Kristian up and inside. I resumed my position and pointed at the hut. We moved forward in silence.

We got him inside and lay him on the floor. The man pointed to the hammock outside and motioned taking it down. We removed it from the tree and as I unwound the rope from the trunk, the reality of my situation hit me. The rope, the empty woods, the lone woman. My hands shook and my heart raced.

He took the hammock from me and rolled it up. He pointed towards the floor where Kristian lay and I moved my torch to where he was indicating. Using the hammock as a pillow, he placed it under Kristian's head. We both stood in the small dark cabin and I breathed a sigh of relief. The ordeal was finally over.

Then the man pointed to something else and again I moved the torch to where he indicated. His trousers were open and he was holding his flaccid penis in his hand. My body exploded with terror and I shouted at him with force.

'No!' I opened the door wide and pointed to the steps. 'No! Get out! Get out now! No!'

He buttoned his trousers and moved towards the door.

I stood, eyes blazing, willing him down the steps. The second he was out, I shut the thin wooden door and bolted it. There were two windows that stood open, balanced on sticks. I looked out before closing them. He stood outside, hands in his pockets, silently staring at me.

The futility of my barrier from him was all too obvious. I went around the small room feeling like I was in a horror movie, hanging towels over the remaining openings so that he couldn't see in, but knowing that if he decided he wanted to there was nothing much to stop him. I sat on the floor for hours in a state of high alert, Kristian passed out beside me.

The next morning was clear and sunny and it all felt like a bad nightmare. I knew how close I had come to tragedy in one form or another and was counting my blessings that I had escaped. Kristian was beside himself, feeling both at fault for the situation and like a failure that he hadn't been able to protect me. He had no recollection of leaving the beach bar and was completely unaware of everything that had happened. It hit him hard. We were incredibly lucky, though. Many others in similar situations both at home and abroad aren't.

In the following years we worked and lived in Bristol, London, New Zealand and Ireland. We were still in our twenties and loved nothing more than exploring country and city pubs around us. English beer gardens with a ploughman's lunch and a pint of local brew. Irish 'old man' bars in the Wicklow Mountains, creamy Guinness dripping down the glass. Pavement wine bars and cool backstreet clubs in Auckland and Christchurch, crisp glasses of Sauvignon Blanc in hand. Everywhere we went, our weekends would revolve around where we would end up for a drink. A walk and a pint. Meeting friends for drinks. Out for dinner and drinks. A wander around a city, stopping in for a beer or three. Everything went hand in hand with some sort of alcohol.

We weren't alone, of course. It was part of the culture everywhere we travelled – or at least we hunted out that part of the culture everywhere we travelled. It never, ever crossed my mind to go out at night and not drink. Alcohol just added something extra to the mix, whatever the situation was. A treat, a reward, a marker, a sparkle.

I was still young and the dreaded hangovers were few and far between, although when they hit they knocked me out for days. Sometimes I would spend 24 hours vomiting up the fun from the night before, but I never considered giving it up. Alcohol was non-negotiable.

At 29, within a year of getting married to Kristian, I became pregnant and we bought a house in the country.

I stopped drinking, almost but not quite entirely. I would sip on a glass of Guinness if we went to the pub, and we did because our social life and friendships revolved around them. I didn't find not drinking difficult – it was those around me continuing to drink that was the problem. One night Eric came to stay over and he and Kristian went out to the local for 'two pints, max' before picking up a takeaway from the chipper. I stayed home and after about an hour began to get hungry.

'How long will you be?' I texted.

'Just ordered our last one,' he texted back. 'Won't be long.'

Time passed.

'Where are you?' I texted. 'I'm hungry.'

'Just finishing up this one,' he texted back.

I could picture them at the bar, egging each other on. 'Just one more ... Last one ... Sure, we never get to see each other ... She's going to kill you...'

They fell in the door hours later, a greasy brown bag held aloft for me. Hunter gatherers returning with their hard-won prize.

I clenched my teeth and poured the contents onto a plate. I was so hungry that the thought of golden battered fish and crispy chips had, for a moment, dissipated my anger.

What slid out of the bag did not resemble what I had in mind. Undercooked chips and a square of fake fish.

'Albino chips and a fucking pop tart? Are you joking me?'

The sorry excuse for my imagined fish and chips feast was not going down well. They looked at each other and fell about laughing. I was furious. Shoving a few uncooked chips in my mouth and throwing the rest of the meal in the bin, I pushed passed them and went to bed fuming.

They carried on drinking, aware only of their next drink and oblivious to the obvious feelings of someone so close to them. Because that's what alcohol does. It reduces your world down to just you and your warped view inside your head. The most important thing is your enjoyment of the night in question, which most often means where your next drink is coming from. Don't let anyone come between you and that.

Last orders. A call to come home. Running out of money. An empty bottle of wine and a closed off-license. A lift leaving too soon. A friend in trouble.

Once you have that magic amount of alcohol in your body, your sense of personal responsibility becomes warped and you put 'fun' ahead of all other choices. You forget about your friend who wandered off at a festival – 'She'll be *fine*!' – because to do otherwise would ruin the now. You go to the party with the weird guys with the bag of cans who you don't trust. You borrow the 50 from your housemate even though you know you only have 30 left for food for the week. You stay at the pub and walk five long, dark, dangerous miles home even though you could have got a lift an hour ago. And you leave your hungry, pregnant wife at home alone while you squeeze in just one more quick one. I know the feeling because I've been there. Many times. You're in the zone, best time ever, golden glow, don't ruin my buzz.

The next 10 years – my thirties – were filled with babies and sleepless nights. It was during these early baby years, full of stress and exhaustion, that the hangovers really kicked in. My body was telling me it couldn't handle it any more. It was too depleted to cope with fighting off the poison. But I wasn't listening. When they were really bad I couldn't move for a whole day. I would lie in bed cursing myself, crippled with guilt and sickness as Kristian looked after the children and I missed out on precious family time together. It wasn't often – perhaps only a handful of times a year – but each time I would promise myself that I would never drink again. One particularly bad day I actually burst a blood vessel in my eye from the force of the vomiting, but even that wasn't enough to stop me. A life without alcohol still seemed like no life at all.

As any parent knows, those long baby-filled days are wonderful but incredibly tough. I spent many hours when the three children were very young praying for the end of the day, when they would be silent and sleeping. That was my time, an hour or two of peace when we would open a bottle of wine and have some quiet adult time. A small window in the day just for me. We went from sharing a bottle on Friday and Saturday nights to finding excuses for pouring a few glasses on a Thursday (almost the weekend), Sunday (still the weekend), Wednesday (midweek bump), Monday (reward) and Tuesday (might as well make it a full house). It was a coping mechanism to get through the days and weeks, but it actually depleted our energy and made the next day even harder.

Then in my forties, there was another major life shift. Kristian and I separated and I became single again for the first time since I was 24. A scary and exciting new world opened up to me and I began to go out to pubs and clubs again. I met new people and went on new adventures. I told myself that I needed this freedom, this new chance at 'having fun'. Best of all, the hangovers were more manageable. On the nights when the children would stay at their dad's house, I would make sure to go out. At first it was so that I wouldn't be sitting at home alone licking my wounds, but before long I was revelling in my new social scene. And the best bit? Without the children there waking me at 6 a.m. to tell me that we were out of milk again, I could sleep off my hangover. I would come to at about 11 a.m., stretch and roll over to grab a couple of Solpadeine, which I would nurse in bed before pulling down my eye mask and lying still until the hunger made me drag myself to the kitchen and then the couch. The children would come back in the late afternoon and join me under the duvet for a movie and, if things were still bad, a takeaway. This was a far more sophisticated hangover than running to the bathroom in a soft play centre to gag over miniature toilets.

But there was still a lingering feeling of guilt, a haze of self-hatred and a lethargy on Monday that sometimes stayed until Tuesday. The deal seemed worth it, though. Besides, there was no alternative. Was there?

Eighteen months after our separation, my friend Rebecca persuaded me to go on a date. Aodhan was a friend of her and her partner, recently separated, into fitness and music like me. It wasn't even a date, she explained, just a group of people going to a gig and he would be there. It was far outside my comfort zone, but on the promise that he knew nothing about the set-up and that the night was just a chance for me to scope him out, I agreed.

I was nervous, so I drank more quickly than usual. I did my very best 'pretend he isn't there' awkward enjoyment, but every conversation felt watched and every move I made felt judged. This was a big mistake. 'But at least he doesn't know it's a set-up,' I told myself. Because that would, of course, be excruciating.

'What do you think?' he asked, nodding to the stage where a young Leon Bridges stood crooning to the much-younger-than-us audience. It was the singer's first gig in Dublin and only those with their ear to the music ground had managed to get tickets. I flicked my hair and mumbled something about it being all right before running to the bar.

It was only much later, after far too many drinks, that I relaxed enough to have an actual conversation with him. We sat at the bar of a noisy pub later that evening, our friends on the dance floor or scattered in corners, and talked for drunken hours about bands we loved and gigs we'd been to. We bonded over Jamie T and I tried to persuade him that The Libertines were essential listening. He nodded politely. Later someone hailed a cab and we all fell in.

The next morning, the sun crept in through the sides of my thin curtains. My head hurt and my eyes refused to open. I knew he was there all the same, though. I could feel his comforting shape beside me. We sat in bed for hours talking about marriage, break-ups, family support and music. Straight to the important stuff. Later I drove him home in a hungover haze, missing his turn-off at least twice and completing a number of paranoid swerves from imaginary impacts before juddering to a halt outside his house.

I should not have been driving. And I really shouldn't have drunk so much. And Rebecca really should have told me that *of course* he knew all about the set-up. But would I have met my future partner without alcohol there to loosen my edges? Who knows.

For the next 12 months, our social life was built around drinking. Red wine at home, beers at the weekend. We wined and dined and went to gigs and bars. All so normal and accepted. My tolerance began to build up again and I felt like I was teaching my body to process the increased alcohol it was receiving. I was delighted with myself.

But even so, whole weekends were still wiped out over a few hours of freedom, much of which I couldn't even remember. A particularly low point was one Saturday morning when I was driving home to get back in time for the children being dropped off. We'd had a heavy session the night before and I was probably still way over the limit. I felt awful, my head banging and stomach churning. I drove on, willing myself to just make it to my house. Please let me just make it to the house.

Reader, I did not make it to the house.

There in the car, alone and shamed, I vomited on myself, liquid from the night before soaking my jeans. The absolute horror. I never uttered a word to anyone about it. Stripping off in the kitchen and sticking the wet clothes straight into the washing machine before anyone could ever know, never to be spoken of again.

Sadly, shocking as it is to see it in black and white, I don't think there is anything unusual about any of this. Close friends have admitted similarly embarrassing tales. We often laugh it off to make it okay in our heads. Many of us are able to pull out certain nights or next days when alcohol made us behave in ways we weren't proud of.

I know I wasn't an alcoholic, even though seeing my history written down like that might make me sound like one. What I do know is that I had become alcohol dependent. I think almost all of us who drink regularly or who binge on the weekend are in fact the same. The thought of giving up seems impossible to us, which is a clear signal that we aren't really in charge any more. If you don't find it easy to give up, then it's pretty clear you're drink dependent.

I also know I wasn't alone in my drinking habits. All my friends and family, through each stage of our lives, drank in the same way. We would share the latest research on how red wine is good for you (it's not) and how Guinness is full of iron (it's not). We would celebrate booze-fuelled nights out and commiserate over dreaded hangovers. And of course we looked down on non-drinkers and avoided them at all costs. I mean, everybody knows that no one trusts a non-drinker, right?

Chapter 2

Getting Sober Curious

In 2016, when my ex-husband Kristian declared that he was going to give up drink for 90 days, I thought he was crazy. 'Why would he want to do that?' 'He won't last longer than a week.' 'He'll become a recluse.' 'Pass me his beer.' I just about understood the Why, but there was no way I could get my head around the How. Like, really? How on earth was he going to do that? For 90 whole days? Madness.

But then a strange thing happened. As the weeks went by he became calmer, more productive, steadier. He looked better. He felt better. He joined a hiking group and spent weekends out in the wilds of the Wicklow Mountains. And he didn't really seem to miss drinking much at all.

Huh. Interesting.

And just like that, a spark of sober curiosity was lit inside me. Not that I was ready myself, just that I saw that it was possible. And that maybe it didn't have to be the soul-destroying, fun-terminating, social suicide that I thought it was after all.

I wasn't the only one who had noticed the change in Kristian. My brother Liam started asking questions about it. He found out that Kristian had signed up to the One Year No Beer 90-day challenge. It was a new website that was being launched in the UK and you got to choose a 30-, 90- or 365-day alcohol-free challenge. Liam is a guy who likes a challenge. He once ran 100 miles through the mountains in Spain just for fun. So he signed up and literally bought the One Year No Beer T-shirt. A new convert.

'How's the challenge going?' I would ask whenever I saw him.

'Fantastic!' he would beam, full to the brim with lust for life. Utterly hateable.

I was a little disappointed. Another one? I could see our family celebrations and Christmas dinners becoming boring, stoic affairs instead of raucous, booze-filled parties. What was happening? And why were they so damned satisfied with themselves? Could it possibly be that I was on the wrong side of the fence here?

The thought kept me awake at night. There was something in this no-drinking lark that I hadn't considered before. I began to wonder whether I should give it a try, but my circle of thought always brought me back to 'not yet' or 'I don't think I'd be able for it' or 'I don't want to miss out on all the fun stuff'.

All the same, I had to admit that I was more than a little curious. So I asked my brother to send me the One Year No Beer ebook he had been banging on about, which I read cover to cover in one sitting.

The founders of the One Year No Beer movement, Andy Ramage and Ruari Fairbairns, are two regular British guys who felt that life was passing them by in a series of hazy nights and hungover days. While they weren't 'problem' drinkers, they wanted more from life and they felt that it might well be the drink that was holding them back. So far, so familiar.

Andy described the end stage of his drinking days: 'Every day had become a slog and some of the enjoyment was fading out of life. My world felt like one constant hangover. I was tired, anxious, just not right at all. I wasn't depressed or an alcoholic; I was just bored with the booze.'

Andy used mindfulness and meditation to break free from alcohol and began researching and studying positive psychology. From that, the One Year No Beer (OYNB) challenge was born.

So I sat with it for a while, just letting the idea stew. I also opened my eyes to other alcohol-free spaces and realised that there was a sober revolution quietly happening all over the world. Articles, books, podcasts, Instagram accounts all talking about alcohol-free living. And they all seemed so bloody *happy*.

What if they were the ones on the right track after all?

A website called Hello Sunday Morning caught my eye. Like OYNB, the focus is on the gains, not the losses. It was founded way back in 2009 by Australian Chris Raine when he undertook a year-long experiment to quit drinking. Chris was a nightclub promoter at the time, so he was really in the thick of it. He blogged about the challenges and successes of his experiment when he woke up hangover free every Sunday morning, signing off with, 'Hello, Sunday Morning!'

I could see the appeal. Whole weekends feeling full of life and raring to go. Wouldn't that be nice. They promised better sleep, weight loss, more money, better relationships, better sex (surely not with all those inhibitions?), a healthier body, a healthier mind. Every piece I read extolled the virtues of this happier, healthier life. But where was the fun?

A recent post on the site from an anonymous writer sums up what a lot of other people seemed to be saying:

> So I eventually realised the hangovers that lasted for days were just not worth the one night (a few hours) of fun. In fact, the nights were no longer even really fun anymore. Rollercoasters are great fun but I imagine if you sat on one for twenty years, the novelty would probably wear off. Not only was drinking no longer as fun as it used to be but it was slowly becoming depressing. I felt like I was walking through a really long tunnel, slowly walking away from the light (the fun times) and into the darkness.
>
> I think a lot of people are under the misconception that a night out with friends was fun because they were drunk. Maybe the night out was fun because you enjoy the company of your friends and they make you laugh.

Hmmm.

But I wasn't yet convinced. I had done a Dry January in 2015 and had hated every minute of it. I'd even written a blog post on it titled 'Dear Dry January. I Hate You.'. In it I'd written angrily:

> *Dry January is a crock of shit. A farce that I have been*
> *stupidly suckered into. Of course, like me, you might*
> *be tempted after all those excesses at Christmas time.*
> *Might think it's just what your mind and body needs.*
> *Well, it isn't.*

But, with all this new information circulating in my brain, the next few months saw my mind in constant debate with itself.

'They seem really happy off the drink.'

'But you tried that – it didn't suit you.'

'Maybe it was just the wrong time.'

'Oh, and just when you've got your life back is the right time?'

'Maybe I should try it again with a better attitude.'

'Social suicide.'

'But potentially life-affirming …'

'You don't have a problem with alcohol. You're not an alcoholic. You just need to work on the hangovers.'

'You're right. Of course you're right.'

My mother invited us all to Sunday lunch. This was one of my favourite weekend activities. We would all gather – brothers, sisters, kids, cousins, exes and boyfriends – and drink good red wine and eat delicious roast beef and home-made Yorkshire puddings. We were a family of wine snobs and would always try to outdo each other with who had brought the best bottle. There would be two on the table, another warming by the Aga and inevitably a selection that would be pulled out from my mother's secret stash in the pantry when supplies ran low. Dinner would be long finished, the kids would be playing outdoors or thrown over chairs in the sitting room watching a selection of screens and we would sit for hours putting the world to rights, reflecting on politics, religion and all those other untouchable arguments that become so important to win when you have a bottle of Rioja coursing through your veins.

This Sunday was different. Kristian wasn't drinking. Liam wasn't drinking. The table was more subdued than usual.

'Well, this is nice,' my mother smiled at us all around the table.

It *was* nice. Different, but nice. We all drank a little less, mindful of how many times our glasses were topped up, aware of the sober souls beside us. We watched whether our voices slurred and how much we swayed when we stood up to go to the loo. Well, at least I did. I can't say for sure whether the other adults were annoyed or put out by this lack of revelry, but the evening finished up earlier than usual and we all made our way home in good time. Full bellies and responsible minds. Monday morning was sluggish but doable instead of a pit of despair that would leave me frazzled for the rest of the day.

'Kristian seems well,' my sister-in-law, Chris, remarked later that week.

'Yeah, he is. The no drinking suits him,' I replied. 'And Liam's still enjoying it?' I already knew the answer. He was sickeningly happy every time I saw him.

'Yes, great. And the best thing about it is, I get his share of the wine!' It was clear that Chris would not be joining him on his sober experiment any time soon.

My sisters were the same. 'Oh, for God's sake! They better be back on it for Christmas or I'm not coming home,' Siobhan texted from London.

I tried hard to work out how I felt about the whole situation. Here were two people in my life that I never, ever thought would give up alcohol, and they were both thriving without it. Then there were the others – the friends and family members who weren't interested in the slightest in taking a break from their faithful companion. Some were even offended that people within our midst had already done so.

What would life be like for me if *I* gave it up? Would I be happier? Because I was pretty happy as I was. Life was good and alcohol wasn't an issue for me. In fact, alcohol added to my life's enjoyment. Considerably. So why would I go without?

By now, months into their challenge, I was still a long way from being convinced, but I certainly started to question things I had never previously thought to question.

Before Kristian and Liam both stopped drinking, the concept of a life without alcohol would never have even entered my head. Drinking is normal. Drinking is fun. Unless you have alcoholic tendencies, drinking is great.

It was the first time in my life that the idea of not drinking had entered my head as a possibility, a choice that someone who was not an alcoholic might make. 'Normal' drinking had always been considered totally fine.

I began to wonder not so much what is normal, but *why* is it normal? Our societal norm is to drink, so it's widely accepted and never questioned. As long as you are the same normal as everyone else, then we're all okay, right?

But why is it normal to begin your drinking career in a field at 15? Why is it normal that our teenage years are spent getting out of our minds on whatever drinks we can get our hands on? Why is it normal to spend every weekend in pubs and clubs and for every social occasion, from christenings to birthdays to funerals, to revolve around it? Why is it normal to need alcohol to enjoy time with friends?

Because that's what we have grown up with. But what if we've all been sold a lie and life is actually better without it?

My brain was exhausted from the constant battle going on. I was curious, but I didn't want to be. I wanted to go back to not thinking about drink and just enjoying it.

I decided to read the One Year No Beer ebook again. In the style of Allen Carr's formula for quitting smoking, I sipped on my glass of red wine while scrolling through the pages. One section talks about what happens when you go out for the night with friends when you are no longer drinking. It begins with the ribbing and jeering – no one is particularly happy that you are ruining their fun. But then a funny thing happens. At about 1 a.m. someone corners you in the bar and starts to ask questions. How did you do it? How does it feel? Do you think I could manage it?

Apparently this isn't a once-off occurrence. It happens almost every time.

Others in your social circle are having these same conversations in their own heads. They are sober curious too or simply tired of drinking. They just need a skinful before they can admit it, even to themselves.

I found myself questioning why I was choosing to drink each time that I did. Was I bored? Or stressed? Or was it that I felt that I 'deserved' a treat? Was I socially anxious? Or was it purely a habit?

The questions went from surface level to much deeper very quickly. Each of those questions had a follow-up question that brought me to another level. If I was drinking because I felt like I deserved something at the end of a long week – a marker that I had made it to Friday night – why was that treat alcohol? Could it be something else instead? How did it make me feel? Satisfied at first, but then tired, then numbed, then exhausted the next day? What if my treat was an early night and then going for a sunrise swim, watching the golden wonder of first light tripping over the waves and into my soul? Could that be a better reward?

If I was drinking because I was stressed, could there be a better way to deal with it? Would talking out the problem or going for a run be more productive than downing three-quarters of a bottle of wine by myself? It would certainly be more likely that I'd find a solution, but it would also mean facing up to the stress and admitting the issue. Easier to just block it out and deal with it tomorrow, no?

And if I was drinking in order to bond with friends, why did I feel like I needed alcohol to do that? Did I feel comfortable with these people? How did we feel about each other without alcohol? Could I go for a coffee with them and still have things to talk about? Then why couldn't I do that in a social setting like a bar?

It's much easier to simply bat away the questions and just carry on as we always have. But it's only when the questioning starts that the veils begin to be removed. Drinking in our culture is so ingrained that most of us never stop to question it at all. It promises so much in such a simple way. Destress, have fun, bond with others, break the boredom, treat yourself – and all you need to do is pick up a glass. No working out what the problem actually is (and then fixing it), no dragging yourself out the door for a 5k run, no awkward social conversations with others. Just raising a drink to our lips. So easy.

The other thing I began to question was other people's reactions to those who choose not to drink. I saw it first hand with Liam and Kristian. In fact, I was one of those people. Annoyance tinged with anger. Why were they ruining everything?

Again, I went a little deeper and wondered why I felt this way. Perhaps it was partly because it held up a mirror to my own behaviour, which I didn't want to see. I was perfectly happy with the way things were going, thank you very much. But now they'd gone and changed the rules of the game. Now I was far more aware of reaching across for that other bottle of wine or how focused my eyes were or whether my words sounded slurred. Now they'd made me question things I didn't want to.

'Would you ever think of doing it?' I asked Aodhan one afternoon as we sat in an ancient pub having creamy pints of Guinness coupled with prawn tacos, the very best fusion of old and modern Ireland.

We looked around the dark bar. Road signposts and old tin pots hung from the walls and ceiling. Despite the sunshine outside there was a turf fire in the corner and very little light entering. It was quiet. A few other couples or friends sat nursing drinks and crisps. It was like a haven from the busy world outside. An escape from reality, a hideout, a holiday.

He hesitated. 'Um, I mean … there are lots of positives.'

'There are,' I agreed half-heartedly.

'But I'd miss this,' he continued, sweeping his hand around the room.

'Yes! Exactly. And nights out. I mean, how do you keep your friends without drinking with them? And what about going out for dinner? It just wouldn't be the same.'

We nodded in agreement and then each stared off into the distance, minds turning.

I believed all of it. I believed that life just wouldn't be the same. I enjoyed my time with alcohol. I loved choosing a good red wine in a restaurant. I loved taking that first sip, the smooth liquid slipping down my throat and warming my chest. I loved the glow of possibilities after the first glass and the cementing of them with the second. I loved throwing worries into the fuckit bucket and ordering a second bottle. I enjoyed the freedom and the adventures.

I didn't enjoy the hangovers or dragging myself through the next day. But that's the deal, right? You have to take the lows in order to have the highs.

Now that my eyes were open to the fact that actual normal people who are not alcoholics choose to not drink, I found myself stumbling on them everywhere I went. Not so much in real life, but certainly all over the internet. Whole communities of happy sober people were patting themselves on the back and joyously explaining to the world, 'Yes, I, too, have been saved!' It's like a weird process of leaving one cult and joining a new one.

'We have all been lied to for our entire lives!'

'The veil has been lifted and I now see the light!'

'I escaped and you can too!'

'It promises everything, but it gives you nothing!'

'It slowly chips away at your confidence, your sense of self, your hopes and your dreams. Until you wake up one day and you wonder what the hell happened.'

'But now I am free! And you can be too! Join us on our enlightened path to sobriety.'

'Join us. Come on. You are worth more than this.'

Okay, not exactly. But the zealous lust for life shown was seriously disconcerting.

I began to follow some #alcoholfree hashtags on Instagram. Some I found irritating, some were definitely not me, but some pushed my curiosity button.

'Drinking isn't rebellious. Not drinking is rebellious,' said @sobergirlsociety.

It made me think. Being the one person in the room sipping on a soda water and lime seemed like the complete antithesis of a rebel. But what do rebels do? They break from the crowd. They don't follow, doing the same thing that everyone else is doing. They forge their own path, going against the flow. Hmmm.

'There's no such thing as alcoholics, just like there is no such thing as tobaccoholics. There are only smokers and non-smokers. There are only drinkers and non-drinkers,' said @holly.

A quote similar to this had popped up in my feed mid-scroll and caused me to pause in confusion. Of course there are alcoholics! Someone for whom alcohol has become a battle. Someone who is controlled by it. Someone whose life is being ruined by it.

But a number of people, including Allen Carr in his book *Easy Way to Control Alcohol*, have argued that alcohol is addictive, and therefore any of us could be addicted – which is really what alcoholism is. So it's not that there are some people who are doomed by their DNA if a single drop of alcohol passes their lips as opposed to the lucky ones who were born with the 'it's okay, you won't become addicted' gene. Any of us could become an alcoholic, they argue.

But as it stands for most of us, *alcoholic* is a word so loaded with negative connotations that it allows us to form an us-and-them construct in our head. Over there are the problem drinkers – the alcoholics – and over here are the normal drinkers – you and me. As long as we're not an alcoholic, we're on the safe side and so there is no need to question our drinking.

So if we're not an alcoholic and we don't have an issue with alcohol, it should be easy to give it up, right? This line of questioning made me uncomfortable.

'Drinking makes you funnier!' screamed another meme. Ha, it *does* make me funnier, I nodded. 'It's just funny how it doesn't make anyone else funnier...' it continued.

Hmmm. Now that they mentioned it, that *was* weird. Other people don't become funnier when they are drunk. They tell the same stories over and over, they get loud and fall into things. And they think they're funny, but...

Oh. Right. Okay, let's scroll on and forget about that one.

Articles started to catch my eye and pop up in my newsfeed. Had they always been around but I'd never noticed them until now? Like when you decide you really want to buy a new car and you settle on a Mini, then all of a sudden Minis start appearing everywhere around you? I looked it up and discovered that this is actually a thing – it's called the Baader-Meinhof phenomenon. And yes, I did start seeing 'Baader-Meinhof phenomenon' everywhere. The irony.

But really, was I seeing all these personal experiences about the benefits of giving up drink filling the internet, papers and podcasts because I was more attuned to it – or because there was a movement going on? Perhaps it was a little bit of both.

Before One Year No Beer entered my life courtesy of Kristian, the only discussion I'd ever had around taking a break from alcohol was in relation to Dry January. Of course there was AA, but that was for those alcoholics over there, not us normal drinkers over here. Dry January wasn't for alcoholics. It wasn't about addiction and control. It was just about taking a break after the usual month-long session that is Christmas and New Year. Sick of drink and with broken bank balances, it made a lot of sense to a lot of people. Millions, in fact.

The first official Dry January campaign was launched in January 2013 by Alcohol Concern in the UK. Four thousand people signed up and from there it quickly gained momentum. It was two years later that I took the challenge, and to be honest I'm still not entirely sure why I did it. Probably like the millions of others I was feeling tired, lethargic, bloated and poor after the holiday season, so it seemed like a good idea at the time.

It wasn't.

I simply wasn't in the right headspace for it. It was exactly a year since Kristian and I had separated. The preceding January had been a nightmare of packing boxes and moving a heartbroken family across countries to try to rebuild a life for ourselves back in Ireland.

I had gone from 24-hour primary carer to co-parent, having to prise myself away from my precious charges even for a night, every fibre in my body wanting the comfort of them around me at all times. But over the course of the year, helped by family and friends, I had found a new life. I wrote at the time:

In one year a seismic shift has taken place.

In place of that shadow there is now lightness and laughter, wisdom and acceptance, strength and understanding.

Part of the shift has undoubtedly been down to finally stretching that unspoken and invisible umbilical cord far enough away from playgrounds, school runs and bedtimes to remember what fun actually felt like.

At first this gentle stretching had to be emboldened by alcohol, but little by little every new extending of the cord, every night out, every child-free hangover, every moment rebonding with friends and family, finally brought me to a place where I can walk out that front door with a click of my heels and not feel that heart-wrenching pull of the cord backwards until it's time to see them again.

This year has seen me sit outside pubs on balmy evenings hearing strangers' life stories. I've headed off on midnight adventures with newfound friends. I've danced wildly and badly in pubs and clubs. I've had shouted conversations across tables filled with good food, old friends and buckets of red wine. I've twirled around Barcelona doused in glitter and happiness and I've bonded with 50,000 people in a field as we belted back lyrics of songs long lived to bands long loved.

*And each time I've come home afterwards, picked up
my 'Mum' hat, and gladly slotted back into my most
important role.*

The same but different.

*You see, it's not that I love my children any less than
before, it's just that I love life more now.*

Alcohol had been part of putting myself back together.
It was my solace on those cold winter nights at home
alone and my joy giver on those fun-filled nights out that
reminded me that I was a person in my own right outside
of being a mother.

So perhaps it was simply too soon. That year had seen
a broken me carefully glued back together. I was fixed
but far from whole. Perhaps I wasn't ready to face the
emotions full on – the loneliness of being home alone
without anything to block out the feelings that I would
be forced to feel. 'The best thing about giving up alcohol
is that you get your emotions back. The worst thing about
giving up alcohol is that you get your emotions back.' So
the saying goes.

Looking back at it now, I think that's what happened
to me. I didn't realise I had untapped trauma still in me.
I thought I had made it through the most harrowing time
of my life, that I'd put our broken hearts back together
and had rebuilt a new me in the process. But in fact, a

huge part of my recovery from my marriage breakdown was avoidance. I didn't sit with my feelings at home alone when the children were with their dad. I didn't process everything that had happened and try to heal my soul. I used alcohol to slightly numb the heartbreak of being the sole adult in the house when I put the children to bed and sat in the quiet sitting room. Not in an alcoholic way, of course. Just in a 'glass or two of wine' way. Just a softening so that I could switch my brain off.

And the nights out helped me to reconnect with friends I had detached from, rather than emotions that I *wanted* to detach from.

And it worked for me. Maybe it wasn't the best way of dealing with a marriage break-up, but it wasn't the worst and it didn't all come back to bite me in the end. So who's to say if it was a bad thing?

I remember going to a wonderful female doctor in the midst of it all for a check-up on my birth control. I was on the Mirena coil at the time, but after four years it was coming to the end of its life cycle and it was time to discuss options. I told her I wasn't sure whether I would need anything ever again. She talked to me so gently about that first year – the heightened emotions, the increased freedom, the finding yourself again, the common rise in drinking habits. Whereas it was all so new and personal for me, she had seen it all before. It niggled in the back of mind afterwards, causing me to pause and consider whether my nights out were in fact a good thing after all, even though everyone else assured me that they were.

When that Dry January came around, I don't think I was quite ready to give up my newfound freedom. Or accept my weekend nights at home alone. Or deal with the creeping feeling that this was what my future held, with nothing available to help me block it out. No wonder I hated it so much.

In the summer of 2016, within the first year of Aodhan and me building a relationship together, he began suffering from stomach issues. Weird pains and reflux-like symptoms were becoming worse as the weeks went by. By September it was bad enough to warrant a doctor's visit. He went to his local GP, who prescribed him some medication and then told him that alcohol could be aggravating his condition, so he might consider giving it up for a month.

That night, he sheepishly told me the news. To be honest, if it had come at any other time in his life he probably would have ignored the advice, but he had become sober curious too. The markers were clearly in place and by the time he recounted the doctor's conversation to me, he had pretty much made up his mind. He was seriously considering doing it.

My first response was one of horror. Our relationship was only a year old and I still couldn't quite believe my luck at having found him. He is kind, handsome, clever and has levels of patience that I didn't know existed. Whereas

I am a single mother of three kids who is just about paying the bills. But in that 'it's meant to be' way, he thinks he's the lucky one.

Up to that point our time together had mostly revolved around alcohol. On the two nights a week that my kids were with their dad, we either went out drinking or stayed in drinking. Tuesday nights were usually TV, a takeaway and a bottle of wine. Friday night was all about gigs, pubs or meals out. After 10 years of being defined as 'Mum', it had been revelatory to discover myself again. Drinking felt like a big part of that. And I didn't feel ready to give that up.

But if Aodhan wasn't drinking and I was, then he might just see me as a drunken fool, talking nonsense and bumping into things. Which would not do at all.

Drinking is only fun when you're in it together. It's just not the same when the other person is abstaining. So what was the alternative? To join him? But then we would both be sober. And – I barely could admit the question to myself – would we have enough to talk about? How would we spend our time together?

The only time in the past year that we had spent a night sober was on our second official date. The night we met and our first proper date afterwards were alcohol-infused sessions. But what came next? I was out of the dating game too long to know.

A friend advised me to spend some time getting to know him properly – no drinking, just talking. I hadn't dated anyone in over 15 years, so I was willing to listen to anyone in the know. When he asked me over to his for a curry the next weekend, I floated the idea of a no-alcohol date. 'Sounds good,' he said without missing a beat.

It was only much later in our relationship that we discussed this obscene curveball I had thrown. 'What were you *thinking*?' he asked me.

'I don't know!' I answered. 'Someone told me to do it, so I did it.'

On that evening we had sat at his kitchen table, awkwardly sipping cans of Coke until it was time for me to drive home. It's testament to his loveliness that he actually called me again after that.

But back to his month off the booze. He must have seen the horror and realisation cross my face when he had mentioned it, because 2.5 seconds later he was continuing, '*You* don't have to do it, obviously. I'm totally fine doing it on my own.'

He meant it, of course. But I couldn't let sober him hang out with drunken me. Who knows what damage it would do to our burgeoning relationship?

'I'll do it with you,' I mumbled.

'You don't have to.'

Yeah, right, I thought.

Chapter 3

The First 30 Days

They say that it takes just three weeks to break a habit. But what about a deeply ingrained habit of a lifetime that everyone else around you partakes in? What about a habit that you're not really sure you even want to break? If you consider yourself a social drinker, a normal drinker, a mid-lane drinker or basically someone who doesn't have a drink problem and isn't an alcoholic, then taking a break for a few weeks should be pretty easy. Right?

To me, 30 days sounded like a life sentence. How would I manage? I committed to writing off the month as a long, boring experiment. I would hibernate for October and be ready to come back renewed for the pre-Christmas social mayhem. My main concern was that I would lose the hard-earned tolerance I had built up over the past couple of years.

Other concerns included being bored, not having any-thing to talk to Aodhan about, my dreaded hangovers getting worse when I went back to drinking afterwards, what people would think, Aodhan wanting to continue longer than the 30 days and him finding out that I'm actually really boring. ('You are,' my sister assured me.)

And then there was the fear that I wouldn't be able to do it. Did I have the sheer willpower to see it through?

When I was about 10 years old, I was deeply religious. We would have family prayers together every evening and Sunday mass was a given. I was a member of the Legion of Mary and during Lent I would go to church every day at 7:30 a.m. before school, and like many other children I would give up sweets for the full 40 days. Sweets were my thing. I adored them. Quarters of Sherbet Lemons and cola cubes, pennies spent on flying saucers and fizzle sticks. I ate far more than I should have and my poor teeth suffered. Giving up that much-desired treat was hard, but it was a good lesson in willpower. Being the child I was, I always took things further, though. I would do random daily fasts from time to time. I think my mother tried to persuade me not to, but the girl was not for turning. At one friend's birthday party I explained matter-of-factly to her mother that I couldn't have any of the party food because I was fasting for Our Lord. I didn't understand the pity and confusion on her face as she wrapped some of the birthday cake and Rice Krispie buns in a napkin for me to take home. Later I laid it all out on the kitchen table and sat there in my party clothes waiting for the clock's hands to move around to 6 o'clock, my self-imposed finish time when I could devour the lot. Daily fast complete. Amen and Praise the Lord.

I was a weird kid.

Now, 30 or so years later, I was about to embark on a new fast. My treat was alcohol and giving up didn't seem quite so straightforward as in those innocent childhood days. I contemplated whether flexing my willpower so solidly through my early years would help. And if not, there was always prayer – after all, He owed me.

But first, I was heading to Amsterdam for one last wild weekend. Aodhan had booked a trip as my birthday present, a long weekend of pure escapism. It fell just after he had been for that doctor's visit, so we agreed we would enjoy our trip and then begin our 30-day sentence.

We travelled over on the Friday and spent the next three days wandering cobbled streets, visiting his sister and her family, strolling around galleries and detouring into coffeeshops and bars. We sat in Hill Street Blues, a famous bar that his sister and brother-in-law helped to manage. It was dark and smoky and the best place imaginable for people watching. Dreadlocked hippies and hardcore bikers mixed with a scattering of sleepy-eyed tourists. We sipped our pints, smiling.

'I'll miss this,' I thought to myself. I didn't want to say it out loud, as it would make Aodhan feel bad – he already felt guilty that he was the instigator of the fateful no-drinking month. But it was true. It reinforced my idea that alcohol equalled enjoyment and that without it our lives would be lacking.

Over the weekend I did what I had done on countless other trips: I drank without questioning it. I believed it added to the holiday. Never in my wildest imagination could I have pictured spending that weekend alcohol free. I would have been depriving myself of all the enjoyment of the foreign break. No way.

We were in Amsterdam from Friday to Monday, and

in a case of truly terrible timing, the day after the trip I had to make an important presentation at work. I tried my best to push all thoughts of it aside for the weekend, but it would pop into my head despite myself, a quick jolt of panic running through me as I wandered around the Banksy exhibition or strolled along the canals. Each time it entered unannounced I would shove it out the door again, but it sat on the curb watching me, ready to creep in when I least expected it.

By Sunday, the anxiety had started to rise. I drowned it with a stiff drink. By Monday, The Fear had set in. Captained by our good friend alcohol, they set sail with a vengeance.

We sat in the airport waiting for the flight home to arrive. My head was sore, my body tired and a feeling of dread had settled in my stomach.

There were two huge leather massage chairs at our gate. We popped in the coins and lay back. The soft whirring and a strong pummelling lulled me to a better place, but there was no denying it. I felt awful. We turned our aching heads towards each other and nodded. We were ready.

We had already agreed that we would stop drinking after the trip, but that morning it was easy to follow through on. A relief, almost.

And so on Monday, 3 October 2016, I began my 30 days on the dry.

I knew that timing was everything. While January is a great time to go dry as so many others are doing the same (and therefore you don't have to deal with so much social pressure), October has its own hashtag – #soberoctober. Sadly, I didn't know this at the time or I would have used it as an excuse.

Mondays, however, are another great time to start. While it can be tempting to choose the first of the month, this doesn't always work out. For us, we were slap bang in the middle of Amsterdam on the 1st of October, so that was never going to happen. So the first Monday of the month seemed like the next best place to begin. Without even trying, we'd ticked off four days before the first weekend.

That October was looking pretty empty socially, which was also a good thing. No way was I ready to take on a wedding, a party or sober dancing just yet. The only event looming large and scary on the calendar was a Halloween charity event at the very end of the month. I tried not to think about it too much, and without admitting it to Aodhan I was pretty sure we'd just end up celebrating the completion of the month a little early. Twenty-six days would be good enough, right?

On Tuesday morning, I woke up sluggish and anxious. The client presentation was my first thought when my alarm sounded and I wasn't sure I could pull it off. All the fears that I'd been pushing down over the weekend bubbled up and I knew I had a clear case of hangxiety. My heart was beating too fast and I felt frazzled and on edge.

Fortunately, the day went well. The event was a success and I collapsed that night in a heap of exhaustion. I'd made it. With that ticked off the list, the rest of the week plodded past unexceptionally. The heavy weekend in Amsterdam coupled with the added work stress meant that not drinking during the week wasn't a problem, it was a relief.

Then Friday arrived. Fridays are my favourite. I'm mostly off work, I do yoga in the morning, the kids are in good form and the whole weekend stretches ahead. There's always a little bit of magic in the air on Fridays, floating around like invisible phosphorescence. You can feel it twinkling over everyone as they make their way through their day. 'It's the weekend,' it whispers, full of promise and delight.

But there was no magic in my world that day. That Friday feeling had vanished. Friday seemed dull, like someone had stolen my sparkle. The weekend still stretched ahead, but it seemed flat, not fun.

Friday night with the kids would normally involve frozen pizzas on the sofa for everyone and a couple of glasses of wine for me. We would snuggle up together, bickering and pulling blankets, to watch some terrible movie inevitably involving Adam Sandler. The only thing missing that Friday was the wine, but it seemed like everything. It's that Friday night feeling. That grown-up moment. That treat that I have earned for successfully making it through another week. Without it, the approaching evening felt like any other night, so I decided to try to inject some fake magic instead. I made homemade pizzas with the kids and bought myself some posh Green & Black's chocolate and a new box of Pukka tea. It was cheaper than a bottle of wine. But it wasn't the same.

Saturday mornings in our house are filled with multiple football runs. I normally dragged myself down to the local club to watch one or both of my son's matches. I'd often be sporting a dull headache and a hit of Solpadeine. I've suffered from headaches all my life. We're a headachy family. As a young child I remember my mother often taking to a darkened room with a cold flannel over her forehead. 'Shh! You have to be quiet. Mum has a migraine,' someone would whisper.

When I was 13, I found out exactly what that meant.

I was going to stay for a night with an American family that was holidaying in Ireland for the summer. We had met them through my father's work and their eldest daughter and I had hit it off. I couldn't believe my luck. She was rich, sophisticated and pretty. She showed me a pull-out photo strip containing professional headshots of her and each of her 13-year-old friends. Every one of them had bright, confident smiles, a touch of make-up and big hairstyles. They all looked at least 10 years older than they were. It was a million miles away from me and my frizzy-haired friends. I had never felt more like the poor country cousin, all hand-me-down clothes and untamed eyebrows. And yet here we were, actual friends, and I was on my way to a sleepover in her new house. Her family picked me up at home and we drove out towards Seapoint, where they were staying. I had begun to get a sharp headache and my line of vision had become distorted, like I'd stared at the sun for too long. But there was no way I wasn't going on this trip. On the motorway, squashed between my glamorous new friend and her equally glamorous sister, I began to feel worse. Much worse. My head throbbed and I couldn't see properly.

'Excuse me,' I squeaked, 'I think I'm going to be—'

'DAAAAD!' one of them screamed.

The next few minutes were a teenage nightmare that I have yet to get over. As the car swerved into the closest garage, the sisters in the backseat with me scrambled as far away from bodily contact as is humanly possible in a 1980s car with seatbelts, clawing at the window to escape. The younger sister stared in a state of shock at her vomit-flecked (brand new) white canvas trainers.

'It's on my shoes! It's on my shoes!' she repeated in a strange sort of strangled mantra, trying to process the horror of what had just happened.

The stench in the car was appalling, but I was too sick to really care. They got me back to their house and put me to bed. I think I've blocked out the rest of it, but suffice it to say that the ordeal still haunts me 30-plus years later.

Migraines continued to plague my family throughout our lives. But it wasn't just migraines. We would also get regular headaches. All of us, all the time. More so than most families. And I was particularly bad, so much so that my hospital-phobic parents took me for a brain scan to see whether there was anything really wrong.

'Has she ever suffered a trauma?' the doctor asked. My mum didn't know what he meant, so she said no. It was only years later that she admitted that I'd rolled off the kitchen counter as a baby.

'Maybe that's what he was talking about,' she wondered aloud. Ya think, Mum?

Anyway, I've been popping headache pills my entire life, so it was no surprise that my head was where my hangovers decided to hang out. Solpadeine was my go-to recovery whether I'd had a couple of glasses at home or spent an entire evening in the pub. 'Hope in a glass,' my sister Siobhan would say. Clink, clink.

That Saturday was different. The benefits had already started to kick in. I felt rested and strangely happy. It was 8 a.m. on a weekend morning and I was stretching out in bed with a smile on my face. Last night wasn't so bad, I thought, and now I've two full days off ahead of me and I feel good! I made buttermilk pancakes for the kids as they eyed me with suspicion and got the boys ready for football.

This time I stood on the sidelines of the pitch, coffee in hand, chatting to the other parents. A friend walked past and stopped for a chat. He'd been out the night before and was now suffering the consequences. There's a strange camaraderie in hangovers. We all know how awful they feel, especially when there are kids to be minded and football runs to do. We feel sorry for our fellow soldier when he's down, but there's a hint of humour too. An unspoken 'sure, I did it to myself' and an 'ah yeah, but it was worth it'. I didn't tell him that I wasn't drinking. For one thing I didn't think he'd appreciate the sentiment, but I also didn't know how to say it, how to explain why I wasn't drinking on a weekend. It would sound clumsy and convoluted. I didn't have the words yet. So I sympathised instead and wished him luck for the rest of the long day ahead. It was 10 a.m.

The day stretched out ahead of me. I'd no plans until later that afternoon, when the kids would go to their dad's house for the night and I'd go over to Aodhan's. So I went to the shops for supplies and spent the day cleaning and baking. Usually I would never seem to have time to get on top of the household chores. As a single parent of three children I was always chasing my tail, trying to be all things to all people while staying on top of admin, cleaning, cooking, shopping and of course a job. It was the usual parental juggle, but with no one to share the duties with. From bins and bills to dinners and lifts, when it came to my home, it was all on me. So by the weekend I was usually too tired to do more than the absolute minimum in housework – a quick run around with the hoover and another load of endless washing.

That weekend was different. I almost took pleasure in scrubbing my bathroom and mopping the floors. The children watched with curious eyes. What was going on here? Was someone coming to visit? We had freshly baked bread for lunch and I looked around the sparkling kitchen and felt like supermom.

But as the afternoon crept in, thoughts turned to the evening and a little grey cloud came to hover over me.

'What are we doing tonight?' Aodhan texted me.

'Nothing, obviously,' I replied, sullen and reproachful.

He offered to cook and we decided to watch a movie. When I dropped the kids off at their dad's and headed over to Aodhan's house, I felt ever-so-slightly nervous. Would this be weird? Would we be able to pull off Saturday night with each other stone cold sober?

'We need a plan,' I said almost as soon as I was inside the door. 'Something to do tomorrow so that we can focus on that instead of the fact that we have no wine for the night.'

We settled on a hike. Which is really a walk. Uphill. But hiking sounded much cooler. Oh God, it was only the first weekend and already I was thinking that hiking is cool. What would become of us?

I sat on Aodhan's sofa in my pyjamas sipping peppermint tea. It was Saturday night.

It wasn't the same.

The next morning we woke up early with autumn sunshine peeking through the curtains. Stretching out in bed, I felt good. Really good. It had been almost a full week since our last drink and the first Friday and Saturday nights had been ticked off the list. The sun was out and all was well with the world.

We made fresh coffee and ate bacon sandwiches in bed, greasy butter dripping down our fingers. I couldn't wipe the smug smile off my face. Later, washed and dressed, we headed up to the woods. The walk took us up the Wicklow Mountains until we emerged on high behind the majestic Powerscourt estate. The light shined out from the edges of thin clouds as we surveyed the lush grounds all around us, the powerful waterfall in the distance below. It was a moment. A penny dropping. A belief that actually, this month might not be so bad after all.

'Pretty impressive,' I said.

'Yep,' he affirmed and we turned towards each other, an understanding passing between us. We could do this.

The next week passed effortlessly. Everything just seemed easier. My mind was clear at work and I was less tired than normal. Home life seemed simpler too. School runs seemed doable and school lunches were pre-prepared for once in my life. I also discovered the bottom of the laundry basket for the first time in a decade.

When the weekend rolled around I hosted a birthday party for a gang of eight-year-old boys and, amazingly, it didn't kill me. I'd also planned a mum-and-daughter outing with my daughter, Kaya. It's something I always promised but rarely committed to, the fear of a hangover often getting in the way. That weekend I knew for certain that there wouldn't be one, so it had been written in permanent marker on the calendar and she'd been excited about it all week. We headed off together and it was lovely. I took her out to lunch and sat watching her on the other side of the table. She wore a pink and grey striped top and denim dungarees, her golden hair spilling down in silky waves. So beautiful. She grinned at me, delighted with this special day. Twelve years old. I wondered where the time had gone. I popped the memory in my pocket, knowing that I may not have had that moment if I had been drinking the night before. Even a couple of glasses would have left me groggy and grumpy rather than bright and overflowing with gratitude. It was a good day.

Of course, not every day was. There were still days that were filled with tantrums, fighting, sickness, lost shoes and short tempers. Normal life had not been magically whisked away. But those days seemed less common and (most of the time) I felt better equipped to deal with them. Parenting is a never-ending cycle of love, pride, frustration, exhaustion and guilt. Not drinking doesn't change that, it just makes it easier to deal with. A little bit of guilt is important – it makes us try harder. But too much and it's just wasted energy. For the first time in my parenting life, my motherly guilt became manageable. Yes, I might have lost my temper, but we're all human and I did take them to the park/give them their favourite dinner/arrange a playdate/bring them swimming/read them stories and a million other things that as parents we do every day. I think it was because I had more energy, more positivity to look on the bright side. So although I had bad moments, I was able to outweigh them with good moments. So the guilt got squashed. Imagine if the answer to the curse of motherhood guilt was giving up drink.

Sundays had now become hiking days. Aodhan and I headed up into the Wicklow Mountains, with or without the children, and set off in our pre-planned direction. I couldn't believe the beauty surrounding me that had been on my doorstep all that time but that I had so rarely visited. It always seemed like too much effort. The weather had been good to us for most of the month, clear skies and crisp air. I felt alive and wholesome marching up the muddy paths and breathing in the mountain air. It's the natural high that is 10 times better than any drug. That 'I can't believe I'm so lucky' feeling that courses through your blood. It's akin to when you eat a really delicious but completely healthy meal. The taste is incredible, you savour every mouthful and you feel fully satisfied afterwards. Your body is nourished, your taste buds satisfied and you feel great. When you eat a really delicious but bad-for-you meal, the taste is delicious and you savour every mouthful, but then you feel like shit. Your stomach is bloated and you wish you had stopped earlier or ordered something else. That's the difference between natural highs and unnatural ones. You get all of the good with none of the bad.

I began to seek out other natural highs. I got up extra early on the weekends and headed down to the sea for a sunrise swim. It was perfectly quiet and the streets were dark and empty. A few lone bodies walked down to the beach, drawn by an invisible force. I joined them. The clouds stretched across the sky in broken strips so that when the world began to lighten, the blues and greys were in perfect symphony. And then the sun came, rising at the curve of the earth. Dark sea, orange light, heavenly clouds. I stood at the water's edge, cold and scared, before immersing myself in the freezing water. The shock took my breath away, as did the world in which I was suspended. Earth, sun, sky, sea, me. For the rest of the day, a quiet calm settled around me.

The weeks passed. I started running more and without trying I began to get faster. I'd been stuck at six minutes per kilometre for so long that I had convinced myself that this was just what suited my body. I had no idea that alcohol could have been slowing me down. I'll never win any races, but I began smashing my personal bests effortlessly. My Runkeeper app was handing out badges like it was a broken slot machine. I'm sure it thought I had been abducted and replaced by a younger, fitter imposter.

My work week became so much more productive. That slight sluggishness we carry around in our daily lives, convincing ourselves it's stress/age/life, simply dissipated into the ether. I had more energy than I knew what to do with.

For the past year I had been in a pattern of drinking on a Tuesday night when the children were at their dad's house. Aodhan and I would share a bottle of wine over dinner and I looked forward to it as a break in the mayhem of life. Sometimes we moved on to a second bottle, encouraging each other on the decision: 'Well, just a glass – we won't have the whole bottle.' Although at times we did. This became the norm. In hindsight it seems like madness. But that's the thing with habits – you don't realise that they are anything other than ordinary until you step outside of them.

Weekends still took a little getting used to. I had no desire to go out to a pub with friends or even a restaurant. What was the point without being able to enjoy a drink? The thought of socialising without alcohol still drove fear into my heart. I told myself all the lessons I thought I had learned over the past 25 years of drinking: I'm an introvert. I need alcohol to relax into company. I won't enjoy being out unless I have a drink like everyone else. Alcohol makes you fun. So I stayed in and focused on the mornings instead.

And it was a good focus. Saturdays and Sundays were spent running, hiking, swimming and doing activities with the kids. And planning. I couldn't stop planning.

Lists began to appear of all the things I needed and wanted to do with my now hangover-free weekends. More time began to open up to me and organising and committing to things seemed much easier when I didn't have to factor in being over the limit or under the weather.

But while the good moments outweighed the bad throughout the month, it wasn't all plain sailing. My sisters weren't happy.

'Oh God, not another one. What are you doing that for?' my younger sister, Maria, rolled her eyes and breathed resentment at me when she first heard I was on the dry. It was the start of the month and I already felt like I was on shaky ground.

'It's Aodhan's fault,' I replied immediately, batting away the judgements. 'And it's only for the month.'

'Well, see you in November,' she said, dismissing me with a wave.

Later, on WhatsApp, my other sister, Siobhan, joined in. 'Boorrr-iiinngg! What's the matter with you all, anyway? You better be back to normal when I come over for Christmas or it will be no fun.'

They chided and bantered between themselves, damning me for my dullness. I'd like to say it was easy to shrug off, but it wasn't. It was all my worst fears being realised. I wasn't strong enough or sure enough of myself to put up a fight. Had I not been doing it in moral support of Aodhan, I may have thrown in the towel before I even began.

Sisters, huh? Who'd have 'em?

(Disclaimer: I have the greatest, most supportive sisters in the history of sisters, so I can only imagine what challenges other people face with this one.)

At that point I decided to re-read the One Year No Beer booklet yet again and join their Facebook group. Just seeing other people's positive stories was amazing. There was Sally, the personal trainer who was the life and soul of every party but who was miserable on the inside. She knew she was drinking too much but was caught in a negative cycle of drink–guilt–repeat. Drinking was so much a part of her public identity that she didn't know who she was without it. She took on the challenge and never looked back, posting daily updates about how amazing she felt and what she was learning and encouraging others to do the same. Or Andy, the down-to-earth guy who thought his life was lacking and realised that alcohol may be to blame. He proved himself right and posted about how much happier he was without it. Countless people who had been drinking way too much and whose lives were spiralling out of control, suddenly on the right track and full of positivity. It was infectious.

As well as my online stalking of the OYNB Facebook group, I was lucky enough to have support in real life too. Going dry for any length of time is easier when you have someone else alongside you, and the fact that Aodhan and I were doing it together made all the difference. There was no need for drink to be in the house, for a start. Going out for a meal didn't involve jealously watching him savour his expensive red wine that paired so beautifully with the juicy steak. There was no dragging anyone out of the bar when someone hadn't had enough yet but you most definitely had.

I also had my brother Liam and Kristian, who were both still off the drink and enjoying life. Kristian was particularly pleased with my bandwagon jumping. 'Stop copying me,' he deadpanned.

In the first weeks of the challenge I also downloaded an app called I'm Done Drinking. It tracked how many drinks I hadn't drunk, how many calories I hadn't consumed and how much money I had saved.

I selected wine as my drink. Half a bottle of wine (three large glasses) is approximately six units. So my usual Tuesday half bottle, Friday half bottle and Saturday full bottle was 24 units a week, well above the 14 'recommended' units.

And the cost isn't pretty either. At €12 a bottle (€96 a month), plus a round in the pub (€30) and a taxi (€20) twice a month, it added up to about €200 every month. That's enough to pay off a car loan, buy new clothes, treat yourself to a weekly massage or facial, join a gym or save for a fabulous holiday. Me? I started a pension. (Who says sober people are boring?)

I learned that there are approximately 600 calories in a bottle of wine, so in a month I saved myself about

4,800 calories. And that's before you factor in midnight takeaways and hangover breakfasts, not to mention the lethargy that goes with it all. There are lots of apps that track these figures for you and it's an interesting exercise to try, but as a medical friend reminds me, on average we underestimate our drinking by 40%, so be honest with yourself!

As the weeks passed, the only thing really lacking was the social aspect. Friday arrived with a disappointed slump of the shoulders. I still relied heavily on alcohol for 'fun' in my mind, but I decided that I needed to dip my toe back into that world before I became a recluse. I went out for drinks with friends and felt awkward nursing my non-alcoholic beer. My friends felt awkward with me nursing my non-alcoholic beer. I think we all wished that I wasn't there.

At the end of the month, we had that much bigger social occasion to attend. Aodhan had been invited to a not-to-be-missed party-of-the-year that was taking place in the grounds of Marlay Park in Dublin. It was an invite-only fancy dress charity event, expertly run by residents of a beautiful home within the grounds. In fact, it was less like a party and more like a festival. The forest was adorned with fairy lights and wooden seats. Well-known bands played on a stage set up in a clearing in the woods. There were entertainers on stilts, acrobats, light shows and fire pits. Free-flowing kegs of beer were nestled in hollows.

Skeletons and circus performers moved around us in a magical mystery land.

We stood awkwardly by a tree with badly painted faces. We had brought a selection of different non-alcoholic beers to try out. It was a pathetic attempt at trying to make the most of it, to inject a bit of 'fun' into the night. But as everyone else cavorted around us, we felt like guilty teenagers, hiding our contraband so that no one would see.

'What have you got there?' a guy beside us on a log called out.

'Um, just a beer,' we replied shiftily.

'There's free beer over there,' he motioned lazily with his arm. 'You don't need to bring your own.'

We sipped at the bottles in silence. The scene before us was undeniably amazing, but we were watching, not participating. We couldn't strike up impromptu conversations with people beside us. We couldn't dance with abandon under the stars. Despite the wonder, we couldn't quite manage to find the magic in the night. At midnight we watched the fireworks display and then agreed it was time to go home. In fairness to us, a festival in the forest in full fancy dress as our first alcohol-free social engagement had perhaps been a step too far too soon.

It was a fun night, but not the lost weekend kind of fun we had come to measure life against. I felt like the sparkle was missing. The magic of mayhem wasn't there. I was just me, with all my inhibitions. Not the shinier, funnier, friendlier version of me that I thought came out to play when alcohol was involved.

It was slightly disappointing. When I tried to work out why, it was because I knew that I wanted to keep going a bit longer on the alcohol-free train because of all the wonderful benefits I was seeing, but I believed that if I continued to not drink, I would be missing out on the magic.

Could I sacrifice one for the other?

In my mind, it was definitely a choice between the two. Were the benefits of time, productivity, health and energy worth the loss of tipsy me? Would I hand over my sparkles for them? The fact that I even had to wrangle with this decision shows the grip that alcohol had over me, and indeed many of us.

With 30 days ticked off the calendar, I had a decision to make. Did I want to try the 90-day challenge? The benefits were obvious, but the losses still loomed large in my head. I would be giving up the magic of the weekend, social inclusion, adult me, fun me.

What I hadn't realised at that point was that drinking does not in fact make you fun. It does not add sparkle to you. It would take years for a conversation to finally change that belief on a deep and personal level.

'When was the last time a friend or family member became a more interesting, funnier version of themselves when drinking?' a non-drinking acquaintance had asked me as we discussed the matter at length. 'After the first?

After the fifth?' It struck a chord and I suddenly realised that my drinking self was not more entertaining and sparkly – it was just my perception of myself that was.

I had always believed that the drinking version of me was a better version of me – fewer inhibitions meant I was able to let loose and be myself. But in actual fact, I am quite introverted and quiet. I prefer deep conversations with a small group of like-minded souls rather than loudly telling stories over raucous tables. I like listening to people and hearing *their* stories. Alcohol wasn't making me more me, it was making me more like someone else – someone I thought I wanted to be. Inhibitions are there for a reason. They protect us. They use our life learnings to help us make decisions. Casting them off is the reason we wake up wracked with embarrassment or guilt the next morning, mortified at what we have done. 'That's not me.' We may think that alcohol makes us a more amazing version of ourselves, but the reality is rarely true.

On day 31 of our challenge, Aodhan and I sat down to talk about what was next. We sheepishly danced around the fact that we had a decision to make: celebrate with a bottle of wine or keep going. Eventually one of us said it: 'I'd like to do it for a bit longer. Will we try another 30?'

It was what we both wanted deep down, even though neither one of us wanted to be the first to admit it. We were both feeling that the benefits outweighed the negatives, so why not?

But another worry rose up in my mind. A further 30 days would bring us into December, and then it would be Christmas. I love Christmas. The whole family comes home, friends I rarely see gather together and traditions all revolve around drink. Meeting the girls for boozy lunches, Champagne and smoked salmon on Christmas Eve, drinks with the family after mass, carefully chosen bottles of good red wine for the five-hour Christmas dinner marathon, G&Ts on St Stephen's Day. I didn't want my precious Christmas ruined, so I pushed all thoughts of it away and just focused on getting through November. We could make another decision then.

Chapter 4

The Mind

The most immediate difference was in my head.

Like most working adults, I had previously experienced what is usually dubbed 'The Fear', a feeling of dread in the pit of my stomach that would start its quiet rumblings on a Sunday at about midday. The thoughts of Monday morning and the week ahead would cast a shadow over the rest of the day, ruining almost half of my precious weekend. I would push all thoughts of it back down as far as I could and carry on trying to enjoy myself, but it never went away. It didn't even matter what job I had. Even when I was in roles that I loved, that cloud would hover over my Sundays, unwilling to leave no matter what I did.

I began to notice the weekends getting better first. The Fear seemed to have taken a vacation and my Sundays were clear and open, ready to be fully enjoyed. Thoughts of early mornings and work deadlines didn't give me that gut punch any more. I was ready to take on what the week had in store. I felt more capable, more in control. Like – dare I say it? – an *adult*.

Within two weeks of giving up alcohol, I felt a mental clarity I hadn't known I was missing. In work I was tackling tasks on a Monday that normally I would put off until at least the next day. Mondays were usually for getting through, Tuesdays and Wednesdays were when the bulk of the work got done, Thursdays were for finishing all the things I pushed to later in the week and on Fridays I took the foot off the pedal going into the weekend. But now, it was different. Mondays became my most productive day, ploughing through big chunks of tasks that would previously have taken me all week. I was rested, revitalised and ready to go after the weekend. My mind was clear and focused and nothing seemed too difficult. Procrastination had left the building and instead I was ticking off to-do lists with a vengeance. I was far more productive than I had ever been. The brain fog that I didn't even realise had been there was gone. Ideas and creativity flourished and issues became easier to navigate. I felt like I was in the driving seat and for once I knew where I was going. Aodhan felt the same – more confident, more capable.

Within weeks, I decided to tackle something else that had been hanging over me. At the start of that year I had signed up to do a Diploma in Digital Marketing. My working life had taken a detour over the past decade. I had started out in the tech industry and built up experience in financial and account management roles, steadily climbing the ladder in big multinationals. But when my children were born I lost my career focus and all I wanted was to be a stay-at-home mum. Over four years and three babies, I dropped from five days to four to three before eventually taking voluntary redundancy. I was delighted with my life, but it was hard work spending every hour tending to my children's many varied needs. I missed using my brain.

So I began to write. First an article for a national paper, then a blog. I had no idea I would love it so much. I met a whole new community online, formed friendships and learned a huge amount without even realising it. It was the early days of blogging and we felt like pioneers at the forefront of something new. We taught ourselves how to use Wordpress and Blogger, how to create header images and snippets of HTML code. I joined Twitter when I didn't understand what it was and Instagram when it was in its infancy. We all learned tricks and tips and passed them around between ourselves. Before we knew it, we were experts in an industry that had never even existed before. We were creatives and digital marketing masters. And big brands began to come calling. I went to a Netflix premiere in New York and got free passes to Disney World Resorts in Florida. I took delivery of a huge 3D TV so that I could write about movies for Warner Bros. I became an ambassador for Lego Duplo and wrote reviews on hotels, games, toys, clothes and more. Soon I was employed by a company to manage their blogger outreach for lots of big brands and to write branded content for others.

Without even noticing, I had built a new career for myself, working part time from home while raising my children. I spent the next five years happily immersed in this world. But then the unthinkable happened. In January 2016, a year into rebuilding my life as a single mother, I lost my job.

Losing your job is never a nice experience. Rejection, depression and fear are all normal reactions to being let go, but losing your job when you are a single mother brings that fear to a whole new level. It's not just your career you're talking about – it's your income, your rent, your roof over your family's head, their food on the table. That's fear with a capital F right there.

I panicked and wept, and panicked and raged. There was much wringing of hands and ringing of friends. And there was, of course, wine. Lots of wine.

And then I took a deep breath and began to make a plan. Although I had been working in the digital marketing space for years, I had no formal qualifications in it. I knew that if I was to find another job I needed to tick that box on my CV. So I signed up to a Digital Marketing Diploma, started pitching my freelance writing and went looking for employment.

By May I had found a new job. A dream job. I couldn't believe my luck. I hadn't completed the diploma yet, but I had paid money that I didn't have to spare in order to do it, so I knew that I needed to finish it. But eight months after signing up to it, I was still limping through the assignments. I resented having to do all the extra work. Between school runs, an office job, home life and general parenting, I had no time or energy left for it. It was falling by the wayside and my window for completion was running out.

Within a month of not drinking, everything changed. It became easy. Every morning I got up at 6 a.m. The house was dark and quiet and I tiptoed downstairs to my waiting laptop. For an hour each morning before sunrise, I ticked off modules and submitted assignments like a digital ninja. With very little pain and effort, I received a Distinction. I know that had I still been drinking, I simply wouldn't have had the energy or focus to do it. The experience spurred me on and made me realise that there were other big goals that I could perhaps now achieve.

The following year, I continued getting up at 6 a.m., day after day, writing paragraphs that turned into pages that become chapters that eventually became a published book. I became an author. It had been one of my biggest life goals ever since I was a little girl, but I'd never thought I would be able to achieve it. I know with absolute certainty that it wouldn't have happened if I'd still been drinking.

I hadn't expected my book to be about the breakdown of my marriage, but after years toiling over a novel that I couldn't quite wrestle into submission, the idea simply fell out of me, fully formed and ready. I had woken with the title in my head and I knew exactly what I needed to do. I picked up a pen and wrote the chapter headings down instantly. I would write the book that I needed to read myself when I was going through my own break-up. A personal account of the emotional turmoil and a roadmap on how to get through. Once Kristian had agreed to the concept, I pitched it to publishers, struck a deal and completed it all in three months. The book practically wrote itself, filling the pages easily, desperate to be set loose.

Seeing the published book on bookshop shelves was a moment of real pride. Not only had I finally become an author, but I also felt like I was helping others to get through one of the most difficult times of their lives. And so my book launch was a very special moment to me, a celebration of the highest order.

On the night of my book launch, I was awash with emotions. Nerves, excitement, pride and fear all jostled for attention. I got dressed up and my friend Danielle, who is an expert make-up artist, gifted me a makeover. I looked at myself in the mirror she held up and wondered who this person was, all those months of 6 a.m. kitchen table writing sessions in my dressing gown culminating in a Cinderella moment. I panicked that no one would turn up, so I texted my close friends for the billionth time for reassurance that at least they would be there. I went through the list again. At least 70 invites had been sent out, but how many would actually bother coming? I divided them into definitely yes, definitely no and maybes. And then the maybes became probably yeses or probably nos. I tied myself in knots trying to picture the room with 10 people, 20 people, 50 people. In the end I gave up and got in the car.

When I arrived at the bookstore there were already a couple of people waiting, some that I didn't even know.

Then work colleagues arrived. Then my friends. And family. Then friends of friends, and friends of family, and people who had heard me on the radio that week. I was overwhelmed with relief and gratitude. Wine glasses were topped up and non-alcoholic prosecco was offered. My sister Maria gave an unexpected speech that made us all cry. I said a few words and caught Aodhan's eye. He smiled back proudly. And then I signed books and posed for photos and pinched myself that this was actually happening. Later, a small group of us headed to the local pub. I collapsed into an armchair by the fire and surveyed the room, taking it all in. At no point had I found myself itching for a drink – not to combat the nerves or heighten the celebration. I was just thankful that I was fully present, knowing that I would remember this day as a key moment in my life. And that going alcohol free had gifted it to me.

Alcohol had been holding me back in so many ways that I hadn't even realised until I stopped drinking it. I wasn't reaching my full potential because my mind and body were spending so much time trying to process the – strong words here, I know – poison in my system. And I didn't see it as a problem because everyone else was doing the same. I wasn't a problem drinker, I was a social drinker. Perfectly acceptable. Encouraged at every turn.

Alongside my personal side projects, I still had my actual job to do and three children to look after. Being a single mum means that there is no division of household chores. From cutting the grass to changing the lightbulbs, it's all on you. Add to that the fact that you have to make sure the bills are all paid plus take on the physical and mental load of family life and you could say that life is busy. Sometimes the stress of it all gets to you. How could it not? But I'm lucky in that I have a good relationship with my ex, and as co-parents I get a break in the week when they go to his house. Most parents don't get any break at all, so maybe in some respects I have it easier.

I remember talking to a woman at a work event a few years ago. Like me, she had three young children, but she worked full time in a high-pressure job and one of her children had ongoing health issues. We got into a deep and meaningful conversation about life and parenting and relationships. I explained my situation to her and how I was recently separated.

'Gosh, that must be hard,' she soothed. Then I explained my co-parenting arrangement and how the kids stayed at their dad's house a couple of times a week. 'So you get two nights child free?' she asked incredulously. 'Well, I don't feel *that* sorry for you!'

And it's true – those nights that the house is quiet are when I get to regroup and recharge. Most parents almost never get that.

But this isn't a competition. Whatever our circumstances, we are all living stressful lives. Work stress, kids stress, house stress, financial stress, relationship stress, what's-to-become-of-me stress. It's all there.

Before I gave up alcohol, if I had a bad day I might open a bottle of wine and have a couple of glasses. It would take the edge off the heaviness in my chest and help me breathe again. When I was running on adrenaline it would slow me down, like the rabbit in the old Cadbury's Caramel ad, saying 'hey there, take it easy' in its slow, dulcet tones. I would happily stop at two glasses. Stress released. Feelings dulled. It was like a little valve, letting out some of the excess build-up of pressure that I didn't need. Once deflated, I was calmer. I'd tackle whatever the issue was tomorrow. But the next day the issue often felt harder. I wasn't in the right headspace for it. I hadn't figured out how to deal with the problem, so I just pushed it away again. Of course, when you do that for long enough the stresses build up and up until they come crashing down on you all at once.

But life isn't stress free. There will always be issues that need to be faced. Now that I was alcohol free, I needed to find new ways of dealing with the inevitable pressures that we all live with.

Running helped, as did weekend hiking. Both Aodhan and I started to explore other wellness offerings now that we had more headspace and more time to dedicate to them. He went on a one-day course to test out the Wim Hof Method, which uses breathing and cold water therapy 'to relieve stress, boost the immune system, increase energy and improve metabolism', according to their website. He spent the day of the course lying on the floor with a random selection of other people doing deep breathing exercises that made you high, then plunging into an ice bath outside in the depths of winter. He came back invigorated and excited. His new routine now involves a freezing cold shower every morning. It works for him.

I went for gentler options. Weekly yoga had been the anchor in my week since my marriage breakdown, but I began to look for other options to complement it. I tried meditation but I got distracted by either inside or outside influences. It's hard to zone out when you have kids barging in and out of your room looking for food, shoes or the TV remote. I decided that any mindfulness needs to happen outside the home. It seemed the universe was in tune with what I needed, because an abundance of options opened up to me. Instagram and Eventbrite were awash with retreats, getaways, courses and workshops on yoga, meditation, crystals, cacao ceremonies, tree hugging and Qigong. My friend, writer Liadan Hynes, calls it the woo-woo club and anyone can become a member. She describes it in *Image* magazine:

> *Every woman needs a woo-woo club. A further branch of your tribe. A group of women who will tell you it's okay, they felt like that too, it's not just you. A*

subtle mesh that weaves around the fabric of your life,
sustaining and supporting you. That creates a life pause,
in which to take down the stress levels.

Sign me up.

I found out that a local yoga instructor was running a weekend yoga retreat on a hillside near the ancient monastic site of Glendalough in Co. Wicklow. It's a valley steeped in beauty and history, and a reverence hangs in the air. I've been going there since my childhood, at first with my parents, exploring the streams, church ruins and ancient graveyard, then later on school tours to learn about the formation in the sixth century by St Kevin. As an adult, I've returned to Glendalough many times, walking down to the lake or hiking the stunning paths above.

The teachers on those tours would tell stories about how St Kevin lived the life of a hermit in a cave high on the mountainside, and my classmates would tell mythical tales about how they had heard that a woman from the village had continually tried to tempt him, so he pushed her off the cliff. We stood in silent contemplation and looked down at the deep lake far below our feet. Splash.

The round tower stretching up into the sky has no doors and only a couple of small windows at the top. We heard how the monks would retreat inside it when the settlement was being attacked and pour boiling tar down on anyone attempting to climb up. I considered the logistics of this suspiciously.

The retreat took place in a tiny village of wooden pods close to the monastic site. Each pod held a double bed and a decking area to the front. The clouds hung over the hillside, giving it a magical air. We did yoga classes in the morning and late afternoon, then ate home-cooked vegetarian meals together at lunch and dinner. Treatments were available in one of the pods and we could choose between massage, acupuncture, facials and reflexology. We strolled through the woodlands, read, breathed and let go.

By the time we returned to our real lives on Sunday evening, my mind and body felt strong and rested. The difference between the retreat and a weekend away drinking and staying up late was worlds apart. I was happy and balanced, ready for what the world had waiting for me.

Around this time, my mother, sister and friend had all been raving about a local lady who does acupuncture. It's something that had always seemed like a waste of a treatment to me. Why pay to get needles stuck in you when you could have an hour's worth of deep tissue back massage? There's no contest. But my mother bought me a gift voucher for Christmas, so I went along. Joan is special. From her sparkly eyes to her knowing nods, it's evident that she's not just someone who does acupuncture. She's a healer. I went into her little wooden room out the back of her house, hyped up on the usual school-run-to-homework-and-dinner-prep stresses.

'My mum gave me a voucher so I had to use it. She thinks you're great, but I'm totally fine, there's nothing wrong with me,' I hastily blurted as Joan nodded and smiled calmly, eyes laughing. Joan knows. We talked for a long time. She told me that my adrenal gland was working overtime. I was basically running on adrenaline. I needed some yin to balance my yang. I climbed up on the bed and as she expertly placed the pins, I felt my whole body deflate. A deep calm settled over me and that night I descended into a deep, deep sleep.

I continued to try new offerings from the world of wellness, scrolling the catalogue from crazy to common classes and workshops that offer healing and restoration. Some hit the mark more than others. My sister Maria, our friend Rebecca and I set up a WhatsApp group called The White Witches so that we could share which hippie club to join next. It's our own personal woo-woo club of three.

A cacao ceremony led by a beautiful American woman promised to nourish the mind, body and soul. We were told to bring our favourite mug, crystals, a journal, a talisman and eye pillows. I wasn't exactly sure what to expect, but it sounded relaxing.

'She better not ask us to introduce ourselves,' Maria side mouthed as we walked into the room with 20 others. 'I can't bear it when they do that.'

We sat in a circle and the host introduced herself before turning to Maria. 'Now, if you could just tell us all a little bit about yourself and why you're here...' I snorted into my empty mug.

We drank cacao, lay back in a sound bath and, horror of horrors, stood to do 'free movement' to music with our eyes closed. I felt like I was in playschool being asked to sway like a tree. My only comfort was that I knew Maria would be hating it a lot more than me. I snuck a peek and it got me through the worst.

The women were lovely, it was a beautiful space and some of the evening was, well, interesting – but it just wasn't for me. Others in the group were fully involved, though, and obviously taking deep comfort from the experience. It spoke to them in ways it didn't to me. Without trying different offerings for ourselves, we can't know which will stick and which will fold.

One that definitely stuck as a humble offering called Soul Society. This monthly crystal and meditation evening in Dublin was becoming our new beloved ritual when the pandemic hit. Soul Society is the brainchild of Dawn Nolan and Merle O'Grady, who were running it without promotion or fanfare for over a year before lockdown in March 2020. It had organically grown into a much-loved and much-needed monthly time-out for its attendees.

The evening starts with a yoga mat, a blanket, some carefully selected crystals and lots of smiles. There's a beautiful guided meditation, written for that night's theme by Dawn. Then there's a little talk about crystals by Merle, the choosing of your take-home crystal, some angel cards and a chance to ask any crystal-related questions. Merle makes crystals magical yet accessible, explaining that there is no right or wrong way to use them – the key is to just go with what your subconscious is pulled towards. There's a short break for herbal tea and cake, then the evening is rounded off with another original meditation from Dawn. The first night we imagined going on a stroll along a clear, cold coastline, followed by relaxation in a big velvet chair by a toasty log fire. It was perfect. Almost like the real thing, but without having to actually get up.

We left later that evening with a crystal in our pocket, a clear mind and a much lighter step. The monthly event became the perfect way of stopping the world and taking some much-needed deep breaths.

Being alcohol free gave me the time and mental head-space to explore all these new things. I learned that there are plenty of other, much more effective ways to relax than a glass of wine or a bottle of beer.

There are two main reasons why I like the wellness route rather than the alcohol route as a means of destress-ing. Firstly, you often get to work through the issue that's causing the problem. Many times I have come back from a run or a yoga session with a clear path of what I need to do to get back on top of life, something alcohol would never have given me. Secondly, I'm ready to follow that path the next day because I have the energy and clarity of mind to do it. If I had sat down for a drink instead, the problem would still be there the next day, like a leaden weight weighing me down.

Falling in love with reading again was another benefit of being alcohol free. I have always loved reading. As a girl I loved nothing more than a Thursday evening visit to the local library, where I would stay until closing time trying to decide between just three books. I would walk up and down the rows of shelves, reading covers and choosing favourites. I progressed from Judy Blume and vampires to the classics, my own teenage bookshelves filled with the Brontës, Jane Austen, Eliot, Orwell, Steinbeck and my favourite, F. Scott Fitzgerald. I thought it was normal, but looking back now, perhaps not. In university I predictably studied English, but found it hard to find the time to read the assigned books. There were too many other things going on, most of them involving the local pub or student union bar.

And so it continued.

While I have always had a book on my bedside table, my opportunities or energy to read them dissipated. I briefly dipped back into devouring all manner of tomes when travelling in Thailand. Three months of absolutely nothing to do on picture postcard beaches will do that to you. I read Salman Rushdie's *The Ground Beneath Her Feet* in a hammock on one of the islands and remembered how magical writing can be. From time to time over the years I would rediscover my love of reading proper books, almost always on holiday, when I had the time and headspace to do it. Margaret Atwood's *The Blind Assassin* by the pool of my in-laws' house in Spain or Donna Tartt's *The Goldfinch* at a little white stone trullo in Italy. But real life didn't allow for such decadence. Real life was exhausting and mentally draining. It was Netflix at the end of a long day and a flick through a couple of pages of something not too taxing before dropping off to sleep.

But as Jarvis Cocker would say, something changed.

Almost as soon as I stopped drinking, my love of reading returned. I found myself ploughing through books instead of taking months to read just one. My bookcase expanded to include more memoir, psychology and politics. With my awakening from the stories that I had been fed around alcohol, I began to dig a little deeper.

Why had what essentially was a drug that poisoned our bodies and minds become so socially acceptable? Was it money? Powerful lobbyists? Were there darker factors at play? In the book *Brave New World*, Aldous Huxley builds a society similar to our own within his self-crafted 'World State'. To unwind and destress, the citizens are given a drug called soma. They line up to receive their dosage and use it as a recreational drug, a measured dose that allows them to drop out for a fixed period of time. It's pleasure and escapism and a cure for any kind of unhappiness. It's the perfect drug – escape with no ill effects. But soon we see a darker value emerge: 'most men and women will grow up to love their servitude and will never dream of revolution,' Huxley writes. Soma is there to keep citizens in their place, which suits the men at the top of the hierarchy who use them to increase their own importance. It symbolises a lack of free will and a type of enslavement. It's pretty out there as a conspiracy theory for modern times – that alcohol is being used to keep us in our place. It's far more likely, of course, that it all comes down to money.

With alcohol's hold over me now broken, I began to wonder what else I had mindlessly sleepwalked into, so I started to read books, blogs and articles I would previously have skipped past. I watched documentaries and listened to podcasts. There is so much to learn.

At the same time, and linked to a lot of the information I was ingesting, I became fascinated by how the mind works. I delved into neuroplasticity, the science of rewiring your brain. The good news is that no, you are not born that way. You can train your brain to grow new neurons, build new pathways, become more compassionate or grateful or happier. It takes work, but the science says you can do it.

But with the good news comes the bad. What is actually happening to our brains when we drink alcohol? Alcohol interferes with the communication pathways in the brain, this time in a bad way. In the short term this causes a loss of control (when you're drunk) and in the longer term can damage, shrink or kill brain cells. The HSE reports that this can change the way the brain works, leading to depression, anxiety, loss of concentration, changes in temperament and difficulties learning new things. This absolutely makes sense to me because after giving up alcohol I experienced the opposite of all those things. I have less anxiety, improved concentration, I'm happier and I have a desire to learn new things.

Studies conducted in both Harvard and Oxford found that brain volume actually shrinks in proportion to alcohol consumed, and that even light drinkers are affected. Harvard Health reported on the Oxford study, saying:

> At the beginning of the study in 1985, all of the participants were healthy and none were dependent on alcohol. Over the next 30 years, the participants answered detailed questions about their alcohol intake and took tests to measure memory, reasoning, and verbal skills. They underwent brain imaging with MRI at the end of the study.
>
> When the team analyzed the questionnaires, the cognitive test scores, and the MRI scans, they found that the amount of shrinkage in the hippocampus – the brain area associated with memory and reasoning – was related to the amount people drank. Those who had the equivalent of four or more drinks a day had almost six times the risk of hippocampal shrinkage as did nondrinkers, while moderate drinkers had three times the risk.

The hippocampus is also affected in the short term, which is why we suffer memory loss and blackouts on big nights out. The immediate effects of alcohol on the brain – like slurred speech and loss of balance – are obvious and evident for all to see, but other effects, such as cell damage, are hidden until it's too late.

If I'm sitting in a bar having a couple of beers with friends, a good feeling will start to spread through me. It's that warm and fuzzy sensation that we're all chasing. It's caused because alcohol releases dopamine. Dopamine is a chemical messenger that is released during pleasurable situations. (Incidentally, dopamine is also released through exercise, music, massage, meditation and food, so there are plenty of other ways to get a hit.)

If I stay sitting in that bar drinking beer, I'll find myself with slower reactions and I'll start slurring my words. This is partly because the alcohol will have stimulated the neurotransmitter called GABA, which acts a little like a tracksuitted Liverpudlian Harry Enfield character that tells everything in your brain to 'calm down, calm down'.

If I find myself 'out out' for the night (which is a much more fun term than binge drinking), then the cerebellum and the cerebral cortex of my brain will be affected, leading me to bump into walls and getting confused as to what is going on because I simply can't process the new information I'm dealing with. I'll start to get dizzy, stagger and I might get blurred vision.

I remember being at the local nightclub with friends one night in my late teens or early twenties. There was nothing special about the night and I hadn't drunk anything out of the ordinary, but I found myself much more drunk than usual and more than I liked. I wasn't sure if I was going to be sick or not, but I knew that I had to get to the bathroom to take some time out. The room was spinning and I just wanted to sit on my own. With great concentration I managed to stand, then carefully placed one foot in front of the other until I made it to the corridor that led to the bathrooms. The mental effort of getting myself there must have taken its toll, because for the remaining 50 metres I ricocheted off the corridor walls all the way down as other girls quickly got out of my way. I may have been too drunk to walk in a straight line, but I managed to remember their disgusted looks as I passed. I get it. I've done the same myself many times. 'Look at the state of her, imagine letting yourself get like that.' *eyeroll* None of us ever mean to get into that state, it just happens all of a sudden. More so when you are young and foolish and knocking back vodka the same way you would a beer.

Alcohol also lowers inhibitions and clouds judgement, which leads to all sorts of situations that we would never normally put ourselves in. From terrible one-night stands to fights with friends, from drunk driving to walking home alone from dodgy parties in dodgy areas, so many people wake up every weekend all over the country and their first thought is, 'Oh my God, what have I done?'

And they are the lucky ones.

This past summer I met up with friends for drinks in one of their gardens. It was a bright summer evening and the house is only round the corner from me, so I didn't bother bringing the car. The roads between her house and mine run close to the centre of the town and at night are dark and quiet. I've spent years walking them home after nights out, not a care in the world.

At about midnight I bid my farewells to the group and headed off through the well-known streets. It's only about 15 minutes door to door. However, walking home that time was very different. I had no alcohol in my system to dull my judgement and I realised that I was very much alone and not particularly safe. I took out my phone and opened Aodhan's number, finger poised in case I needed to make an emergency call. I checked behind me and although there was no one there, I walked faster. And then a man emerged from a road to my right, a dark, imposing figure in the quiet night. He looked over. I looked away, finger ready, steps quickening. He turned the corner and walked the other way. I rounded the bend and a streetlight came into view. I checked over my shoulder once more, then let myself breathe for the 5-minute home stretch. I was fully aware of everything around me, what could happen and what I might need to do if it did. If I had been drunk on that walk home (as I had been many times before), I would have been blissfully unaware of any danger, but also unprepared and unprotected too. These are the walks young women take night after night, alone on our roads.

It's not just about the immediate effects, though. The long-term implications of drinking on the brain are frightening. Most of us know (and laugh about) the fact that alcohol kills our brain cells, but brain damage, brain fog and changes in personality are also very real results from drinking too much over long periods of time. Often we're so used to the feeling of that slight mental fogginess that we live with that we don't even notice. Stopping drinking felt like my brain went through a washing machine and came out all clean and fresh when I hadn't even realised it was cloudy and soiled. The good news is that damaged regions of the brain can regenerate when we stop drinking, although it can take months to heal properly.

Some of the most frightening information around the mind and alcohol is when you look at the teenage brain. From the age of 12, children's brains are reforming, rebuilding, being coded into formation – ready for adulthood. It's like a building site and everything that goes into it makes the foundations either strong and secure or shaky and uncertain. Problem-solving, learning capabilities, processing complex information and future-planning are all formed and developed during this time. Drinking alcohol disrupts this process. It is now understood that the teenage brain is more likely to become addicted to alcohol than the adult brain. The HSE advises that teenagers who drink before the age of 15 are more likely to misuse alcohol in later life. This type of information is only now trickling through to the public domain. Has it been hidden up until now or were we just not ready to hear it?

I don't know if it has anything to do with my teenage drinking, but I've had low-level anxiety attacks for years, although I didn't really put a label on it for a long time. I simply didn't understand what it was.

The first time I experienced it, I was in my late twenties at a boardroom meeting. It was a group of people I felt comfortable with and there was no direct pressure on me to speak or perform, but midway through I felt my heart quickening and a distinct need to get out of the room. I couldn't focus on what was being said as I tried to figure out how I could excuse myself to get out the door to my left. It was all I could think about. I began to get a little lightheaded, which made me panic that I might faint and then fret about how embarrassing that would be, which made my heart race even more.

From then on, every time we had a meeting in that room I would be on edge, wondering whether the feeling would come back again. When we had whole-company gatherings in there, I would place myself by the door for easy access, just in case. A couple of times I had to excuse myself when I felt the rising tide of anxiety wash over me.

Large, quiet gatherings became my nemesis. Whereas I was fine in a noisy pub or restaurant (could it have been the alcohol?), churches were a no-go. I stopped going unless it was absolutely necessary. I dreaded funerals, and Christmas Day mass became a thorn in my side on an otherwise perfect day. At my niece's confirmation in London, where I was there as her sponsor, I dug my hands into the rail in front of me, trying to count my breaths so that I didn't make a scene. I pictured what would happen if the anxiety got worse and turned into a full-on panic attack. What if I fainted? I couldn't bear the idea of ruining her day and turning all the attention on me. Being the centre of attention is not my scene at the best of times, but it was 10 times worse when it was supposed to be on my lovely niece. I leaned towards my sister and whispered, 'I'm feeling a bit panicky.'

I had heard that telling someone takes some of the power away from the feeling, as you're not on your own, there's someone else there looking out for you. Being well versed in mental health issues, she whispered back, 'Use your senses. Concentrate on what you can touch, hear and smell.' I did as I was told, but it made no difference. I bore it until we were released outside and all tension evaporated into the sunshine, carried away on the breeze. It frustrates me that something that is nothing can ruin a special occasion like that. I'm at its mercy and it can come and go on a whim.

For years, I got by using avoidance. Quiet gatherings make me anxious, so I avoided quiet gatherings. After my separation, however, which involved a traumatic international move from Spain to Ireland, and a fear of the future that was total and complete, I was struck down when I least expected it. The break-up had happened, as is so often the case, in the aftermath of Christmas. We were living abroad in a last-ditch effort to rebuild our family, but it hadn't worked out. The next six months were achingly painful emotionally and financially, but with lots of support I had clawed my way back to some form of stability. I had a house and a part-time job. The kids had been welcomed back to their old school and friend groups. We had made it through the worst and we were okay. Now it was the summer holidays and we could all relax and recover.

The sea is my safe place. Whether swimming in it or walking by it, it always centres me. Which is why I was thrown so utterly off guard when I felt the first flutterings of anxiety rising up in my chest that day. The sun was shining, the beach was busy, the children were all playing happily and moments before I had felt content and hopeful. Anxiety had no place there. And yet. I got through it, silently talking myself to the other side. But it frustrated me.

I honestly can't recall if I had been drinking the nights before these incidents, but it was certainly a standard part of my life over those years. The improvement in my anxiety after giving up alcohol wasn't immediately evident, as

I could go months without it visiting. Over time I have learned to identify the first flushes of the attacks – a quickening heartbeat or the feeling of something bad looming – and am able to talk myself down. But after a few months I realised that those moments hadn't arisen at all. Perhaps I need to find a funeral to test myself out on.

Apart from anxiety issues, there are, of course, other challenges to face, both in work and life in general, but I feel far more able to take them on now. The ungrounded fear has left me – I can see the problems and stresses for what they are, nothing more and nothing less. I'm not trying to escape from them through drinking and I'm not building them up to be more than they are due to the after-effects of the drug being in my system. I see them, acknowledge them and deal with them in the best way that I can. I still get troubled and worry when one of the children is going through a hard time and I still get disappointed if something doesn't come off as planned in work, but I don't waste precious time and energy worrying about things that may never happen. Momentum is continual, which I've discovered is the key to progress in every area of our lives.

The irony is that for years I believed alcohol helped to make me feel less anxious. Social anxiety was quashed almost instantly using it. Stressful days were put to bed with a cold beer or a glass of wine, drawing a line under the difficult part of the day and marking out some down time.

But the fact is that the exact opposite is true. Drinking compounds stress and anxiety.

According to the Verywell Mind website, alcohol causes higher amounts of cortisol to be released, altering the brain's chemistry and resetting what the body considers 'normal'. Alcohol shifts the hormonal balance and changes the way the body perceives and responds to stress. Alcohol prevents the body from returning to its initial hormonal balance point, forcing it to set a new point of physiological functioning.

Further, the Healthline website states that alcohol changes levels of serotonin and other neurotransmitters in the brain, which can worsen anxiety. It essentially just presses a pause button on the problem, which comes back even stronger once the alcohol wears off.

Many of us use alcohol to either heighten or dull our emotions. We use it to escape the stress of a bad day, to dull uncomfortable feelings or to make a happy occasion even happier. The problem is that it doesn't work. Like with anxiety, alcohol only impacts the emotion for a short period of time. If we're drinking to escape our feelings of low self-worth caused by a bad relationship, to dull the pain of being stuck in a dead-end job, to block out the unhappiness caused by feeling like you aren't where you're supposed to be at this stage of your life, to lessen the frustration of dealing with teenagers or toddlers all day, to ease the guilt of being a 'bad mum' that day or whatever it is that life throws at each and every one of us, then the only things that are certain is that alcohol won't help us deal with that emotion or improve our situation. We need to get used to *feeling all the emotions*, which can be incredibly hard for some of us.

Some people begin to get caught in a trap. They started drinking to feel good, but as time goes on they find themselves drinking to stop feeling bad. If you've ever taken a drink because you're stressed, unhappy, anxious, worried or angry, then this is you (and me).

While drinking might make us feel good for a moment – whether it's to escape or to celebrate – without fail, along comes the morning after and with it the hangover blues. One night when I was very young, my mother drank too much wine (probably homemade). The next day she had a horrendous hangover. Head banging, eyes hurting, she sent us packing off to friends' houses. My sister skipped up the road to her best friend's house, whose parents happened not to drink at all. (Teetotallers! Unheard of!) 'Mummy got alcoholic poisoning,' she announced with a serious face. Whether she was worried about our mum or just getting revenge for being sent out of the house, I'm not sure, but my mother spent the next two weeks hiding behind the garden wall whenever the parents passed by. Poor Mum. It took her years to get to the laughing-about-it stage.

I grew to know that feeling well, that awful moment when you wake up and you know it's going to be a bad one. And I have had many, many bad ones.

When I lived in Australia, I drank a lot. The Aussies like their booze as much as the Irish – no wonder we get on so well. One morning I woke up in my flat, sunshine streaming in through the shutters, the golden beach waiting for me at the end of the road. But I was more interested in making it to the toilet. I dragged myself out of bed, stood up and out of nowhere the floor rose up to whack me in the face. I'd never experienced anything like it. I stumbled back to the bed, whimpering. For my second attempt, I crawled instead.

Most of the effects of alcohol on the brain – splitting headaches, dizziness and confusion – are avoidable if the liver is able to process the amount you have ingested. But when you drink too much, your body literally can't cope with the poison you have put into it – and so you suffer.

Alcohol causes your blood vessels to expand. As the alcohol wears off, the blood vessels begin to contract. Both the expanding and the contracting cause your head to hurt. Dehydration makes you dizzy. Disrupted neurotransmitters make you ultra-sensitive to light and sounds. Your brain is screaming and you are filled with regret. Never again.

Chapter 5

The Body

My first stop when I landed in Australia, in my mid-twenties and all alone, was to visit my childhood best friend on the Gold Coast in an idyllic town called Noosa. Jenny and I had grown up together. We lived in the same town, went to the same school and had the same obsessions at the same time. What more do you need from a soulmate? Jenny had blonde hair and blue eyes and was the polar opposite to my black and green. Over the years we built dens, had sleepovers, played basketball, went on diets, kissed boys and had our first drinking experiences together. (She was also the other half of the earlier hospital brain scan escapade.) We lived in each other's pockets until we were 16 and in our final year of secondary school.

'You have to promise not to tell anyone,' she said as we walked back home from the sea one evening, taking slow steps over the old iron bridge. You always knew it was going to be a good story when it started like that.

But it wasn't a good story. It was a terrible story. She told me that her family was thinking of moving to Australia, and I knew by the way she said it that it was going to happen. My world crumbled and I lived in denial for the next few months.

When they left, we both cried. This was pre-internet, pre-mobile phones, pre-Facebook and pre-email. We would write long letters to each other on impossibly thin airmail paper, blue like the sky she was taken away in. I would gather with her other friends and we would make tapes of us talking rubbish until we ran out of recording time, 45 minutes on one side and 45 on the other. Ninety minutes of pure teenage nonsense. She loved it. About two years after moving continents, Jenny found a broken phone box in her new town and would queue to make hour-long calls to me. I'd sit on the front doorstep of my house, pulling the telephone cord as far as it would go to gain some privacy and sunshine.

And now, almost 10 years later, I was finally going to see her again. I stepped out of the airport minivan just in front of her house. I was overweight, pasty winter white and wearing an oversized hoodie and combat trousers. Jenny danced down the wooden steps in her bare feet, her golden skin and toned body rushing towards me. My joy at seeing her was mixed with horrendous jetlag and a massive dose of country cousin-ness. Her partner followed her out, similarly tanned, fit and healthy looking. I wanted to run away and come back after losing two stone and spending three months browning myself.

It turned out that the new Jenny was a bit of a health nut. She and her chef boyfriend ate only organic vege-tarian food. They drank vats of (room temperature only) water every day. And they didn't really drink alcohol. They talked about blood type diets and the raw food revolution. This level of health knowledge was unheard of at this time and I was horrified and enthralled in equal measures. Her eyes sparkled and her skin was clear and bright.

I wanted to be like Jenny.

I spent three weeks at their home, reconnecting with my old friend and learning new ways of living. I was fascinated by the clarity of her eyes – no one I knew had eyes like that. I was so used to looking at slightly cloudy versions that I thought that was just the way adult eyes were. You lost that wide-eyed wonder of childhood. But Jenny's eyes told a different story.

Not that I was ready to try giving up or even cutting down drinking at that stage. After my time at their home, I left to go to my first Australian hostel, where I met Kristian, got drunk, then spent the next decade with decidedly non-sparkling eyes.

But within days of my 30-day challenge, I found that I looked better. 'Take a picture on day one,' I was told, then compare it after 30 days. I didn't need to. I saw the difference every day when I looked in the mirror. Within two weeks my eyes had found their sparkle again.

Aodhan has blue eyes. The first Christmas after we stopped drinking, my sister Siobhan was home from London. 'Oh, wow!' she remarked as we came in and sat down. 'Your eyes are so blue! I've never noticed them before.'

Of course she had never noticed them before. They'd been dulled and clouded like everyone else's. It's amazing the impact that alcohol-free eyes can have on you when you get to actually appreciate them. (They're pretty good looking out from the other side too.)

Why does this happen? When you stop drinking your eyes actually become brighter and whiter as your body counteracts the damage to the sclera (the white part of your eye), which may previously have been dulled or tinged yellow from drinking. Added to this is improved circulation, meaning our eyes receive more oxygen and nutrients. This leads to the disappearance of irritation and dry eye. It's no wonder they are so happy and sparkly. It takes less than one month for liver health to improve when you stop drinking, which is reflected in the condition of our eyes. They are the windows to the body as well as the soul.

It wasn't long before the compliments started coming.

'Did you get your hair done?'

'Did you change your make-up?'

'You look so *well*!'

I could see it myself. My skin was brighter, more glowy. Like when you're on holiday and the stresses of life have drifted away and daily naps are the only task on each day's agenda.

A colleague opened the door for me as I arrived at work on a Monday morning. 'You look great,' she said suspiciously, eyeing up my face for clues. 'New foundation?' I'm pretty sure she thought it was Botox.

One of the biggest effects that alcohol can have on your skin is the dehydration it causes. Wrinkles and pores become more visible when your skin is dehydrated. You lose plumpness and elasticity. Alcohol can also cause inflammation, meaning that you get that lovely blotchy face and ruddy cheeks after a session. Add in puffy eyes and broken capillaries and it's a wonder our vanity allows us near the stuff.

The good news is that it only takes about a week to begin to see the difference. Within a month you will be glowing again. It's more effective than any expensive anti-ageing serum and – bonus! – it actually saves you money too because you are not buying the very thing that is causing the ageing problems in the first place.

The changes weren't just on the surface either. One of the key differences in giving up alcohol for 30 days this time as opposed to that fateful Dry January was my change in mindset. Instead of focusing on loss and deprivation, both myself and Aodhan were now looking for the gains. What were the good things we could take from this experience? My brother Liam told us to sign up for some sort of fitness challenge. It didn't matter what it was, it just had to be a little beyond our current capabilities.

I like a good fitness challenge. I was always sporty in school, swimming and basketball being my two great loves. Summers were spent diving off boards and bridges into the freezing sea or hanging around the school basketball courts until it was too dark to see the hoop. In college I would do laps of the campus pool and in my early twenties I became a gym addict.

I fell off the fitness wagon during my travelling days and didn't really think about it again until after my third child. Unlike most people, my weight had actually gone down after having children (don't hate me). Extended breastfeeding meant that it had fallen off. I could eat what I wanted without putting on the pounds, so why would I bother exercising?

Some of the other local mums had decided to start running. I went out with them for a couple of evenings and was shocked at how unfit I was. My chest burned and my mouth watered. Every time I had to stop and walk, I felt like a failure. But I persisted, driven on by the 10k Women's Mini Marathon that some of us had signed up to in support of a good friend who had recently lost her son in a tragic accident. I would think of him as I slowly jogged through woodland trails and down winding roads.

After that first year, we did the event every year. I would stop running almost immediately after the event, then start up training the next year just in time to make it round the course. I was slow, but every year I came in around the one-hour mark. I was pretty sure that meant that this was my natural speed: 10k in 60 minutes. The same every year.

So when I signed up to my alcohol-free challenge, a 10k Run in the Dark in Dublin in November, I expected the same thing. But as I trained for it, I found myself getting faster. I wasn't trying harder or doing anything differently,

I simply felt lighter and fitter. On the night of the run I waited nervously in the crowd, ready to be set free into the streets. And then we were off. I lost Aodhan in the crowd early, but continued the run on my own. It felt almost effortless. I came in smiling and happy before seeing my time: sub 50. My fastest and most enjoyable run ever.

Over the next few years, I kept running. I did it for my head and my body. I mostly stayed around the 10k mark, rarely if ever going over that. But there was something that I had always wanted to do.

'Anyone can run a marathon,' someone had told my dad when I was about 10 years old. 'You just need to train for it'.

And so he began. He started off running on the spot in his bedroom for 10 minutes a day because he didn't want to have to stop on the road in public. Slowly he built up the miles pounding the pavements. This was the 1980s. There were no headphones, no music, no running apps, no gels, no flashy gear. Just him, an old pair of shorts and the Wicklow Mountains. There were times he got caught 10 long miles from home in the driving rain in the depths of winter. With no phone and shivering cold, he found an old bin bag and put it on, thanking the heavens for saving his life. He ran home and up through the town in it. 'Is that your dad?' a friend asked my older sister, a teenager at the time. 'Never seen him before in my life,' she quickly responded as a cock crowed three times in the distance.

Dad went on to run the Dublin, Belfast and Boston marathons. We all thought he was mad, but secretly I was very proud of him. It always stuck with me, his journey from zero to hero. And I always wanted to run one too. It just felt too long and too scary. An impossible feat.

Until I gave up drinking.

Suddenly, scheduling long runs on the weekend didn't seem impossible. I wouldn't be drinking, so I wouldn't be hungover, so there was no excuse. I could also get up early on the weekdays, as I had previously for my other big goals.

So when an online friend shared the entry link, I took a deep breath and signed up. The fear was very real and I immediately texted any person I knew who had run a marathon before. 'Pick a plan and stick to it' was the advice I got. And oh my God, did I stick to it. I was terrified that if I strayed from the training schedule all my hard work and resolve would disintegrate around me, so for 20 weeks straight I ran five times a week, clocking up over 500 miles.

Each day I would set the alarm for 6 a.m., drag myself out of bed, head off in the dark and run uphill for 3 miles and back for 3 miles. Then on the weekend I would tackle the long ones, 8 miles, then 10 miles, then 12 miles, then 15 miles, then 18 miles, then 20 miles. I felt superhuman.

From the little girl aged 10 who had heard those fateful words that 'anyone can run a marathon' to the middle-aged mother of three who knew she had it in herself to complete one, the marathon really was the challenge of a lifetime. When the day of the 2019 Dublin City Marathon dawned, it was bright, clear and sunny. The stars had aligned for me. But I was nervous. More nervous than I have ever been. All that training, all those early mornings, all those tired muscles and hours on the road – what if I didn't make it? What if I got injured? Or ran out of steam? Or had to walk the final stretch?

What if I disappointed myself?

The crowds of runners milled around me and my nerves increased. I needed a last stop at a Portaloo. The problem was, so did everyone else. I joined a long queue, checking the time continuously. I couldn't miss my start.

I missed my start.

I had planned to head off with the four-hour balloon marker, but by the time I ran out of the toilet, he had already gone. So I ran to catch up. This was not part of the plan. As my breathing deepened and my stress settled, I gave up the race to catch him and started to enjoy myself. The other runners, the unbelievable number of supporters, the music, the sights. Through the centre of Dublin, round Phoenix Park, out west, then south. I had no idea where I was going as I followed the crowd, but I was enjoying it.

'Katie!' someone shouted as I ran through Crumlin. My friend Emma stood at the side of the road smiling and clapping. I grinned back and kept running, hitting 'tap to power up' signs held by children as I went.

'There she is! Mum!' My daughter, Aodhan and my sister Maria stood at the bottom of the hill as Dexys Midnight Runners' song 'Geno' spilled from the speakers. I thought my heart might burst. The queen of refusing high-fives stuck up her arm and smacked hands with each of them as she passed.

At 15 miles the running app on my phone decided to stop working, meaning I had no idea of my times. Distance, duration, minutes per mile were all lost to me as I ran the next 11 miles. I never did seem to catch the elusive four-hour balloon. Time had lost all meaning. But it didn't matter any more. I was doing it. A massive life goal was being ticked off my list and I was high on life.

As I neared the end I could see the red balloons of the finish line in the distance. This was it. I put in a sprint finish but then realised that they weren't actually the finish line. Never mind, there's the next set – that must be it. I sprinted again but no, just more balloons.

And then there it was, the undeniable finish line. I gave one last push and raced over the line. I checked my time at the first opportunity – 3:58:59. I had made it in a dream sub-four-hour time with seconds to spare. I walked up to meet my little band of supporters, medal swinging from my neck. It was one of the proudest moments of my life. And I achieved it only by giving up something that I had thought was helping me to live my life to its fullest.

I also started dipping my (freezing) toe into year-round sea swimming. The summer of that first year of no alcohol had been full of warm days and frequent dips in refreshingly cold water, but as the clouds ushered in the autumn, it didn't seem quite so inviting. Even so, during that first month of going sober I decided to do some sunrise swims. There was a small group that met at the cove every morning. Some I knew from around the town, some I knew simply from their beautiful Instagram photos. Very occasionally I would join them. The Happy Pear twins brought spicy tea and healthy snacks and offered them around. It was a beautiful community vibe that I stood on the edges of. Some of the swimmers would spend what felt like hours just floating and chatting in the icy water. I took 10 quick strokes and picked my way up the stones with painful feet, skin tingling, body shaking. But the vision of dark skies turning pink, purple, red and gold over a sea that touched the edge of the world was more than worth it. You couldn't help but marvel at the vastness of the universe and the smallness of our own bodies and lives. It was a meditation in and of nature that grounded me for the rest of the day.

I've always been a fair weather swimmer, but I now set myself the challenge of at least one outdoor swim a month. Initially it was sunrise swimming, but as the months went on I would cherry pick my days depending on the weather or if I had been for a run. The feeling of diving under freezing waves after a long run will never be anything less than glorious.

For the next three years, I didn't miss a month. Over that time I discovered that I preferred swimming alone, so I moved to a quieter shore. And then something unexpected came along, something none of us could have predicted. In March 2020, the announcement of the school closures due to Covid-19 pulsed through the airwaves, allowing no room for any other thoughts. In a matter of seconds, everything shifted. The world ceased to turn while we held our collective breath. It seems apt that the dawn of the next day was Friday the 13th.

The days that followed were filled with an onslaught of information – messages, classes, emails, WhatsApp messages, phone calls. How to work from home! How to make sourdough! Free crafting classes! Instructions for First Years! And Third Years! And Fifth Class! How to use Dropbox! How to volunteer! Store opening times! Free PE! Primary school books! Secondary school resources! New government announcement! And a billion memes.

So. Many. Memes.

So overwhelming.

I dove into the freezing sea on the morning of Day One, washing the unwanted party of thoughts from my head and resetting my system. It brought calm and clarity and a new addiction was born.

Every morning I now set my alarm for 6 a.m., have a coffee and then head down to my favoured swimming spot. In fact, as I write this I've just returned from today's swim. It's a grey July day but there is always a small group gathered. Men and women in wetsuits, lone dippers, goggled-up swimsuited skin swimmers. This morning a couple came down the steps with what looked like a kit bag. It took a moment to realise that it was a car seat that he was carrying, a tiny newborn sleeping in it under blankets. New parents searching like the rest of us for that headspace, that body shock, that start to the day that would make it a good one.

I swim more than 10 strokes these days. My body acclimatised, I head off down the beach to the lifeguard hut, the blue flag or if I'm feeling particularly good, the first arch. My body feels fit and strong and my mind feels clear.

I've wondered more than a few times how life would look at this moment in time if I was still drinking. So many people have used alcohol as a crutch to get through the uncertainty of these past few months. It's undoubtedly been a struggle, but while alcohol helps to release the anxiety and pressure for that evening, it hinders progress in the long term. More pressure, more alcohol. I know a lot of people who have been caught in the daily drinking cycle. They are now questioning their routine but finding it hard to break free from it. It's understandable. I was caught in that cycle myself when my children were young.

Sea swimming isn't for everyone, but I am so grateful that my crutch during this time is a wholesome one. It's one I don't think I would have found if I was waking up groggy and tired, a couple of glasses of wine from the night before still in my system.

I've always been the annoying early rising, outdoorsy type. When I was in my late teens I would generally be up and out on the weekends whenever I got the chance. One Sunday morning I called into a friend's house and some of our gang were already there. It was coming up to midday and conversation had turned to food.

'Will we go out for breakfast?' Avril asked.

'Breakfast? It's almost lunchtime,' I said.

'Look, Katie. I know you've probably been on a 10k hike up the mountains already, but some of us are just getting to grips with the day, okay?' Aoife countered, holding her head and knocking back a couple of paracetamol.

And the funny thing was that I had. I'd dropped in on my way back from climbing the Sugar Loaf mountain, full of the joys of windswept endorphins. What a pain.

But over the years, the mountain walks had become less frequent. Weekends began to revolve around kids' activities, and walking with three unhappy toddlers or tweens moaning about being tired and wanting to go home simply didn't have the same *joie de vivre* about it. The weekend days of the kids' early years were more about sports runs, playgrounds and catching up on household chores, and the nights were relaxation time – dinner, movie, wine, treats. That's the way it was for years and would have continued indefinitely.

Now, though, I have been given a chance to reclaim my love of the great outdoors. Aodhan and I began to explore the Wicklow Way and the abundance of stunning walks right on our doorstep.

As the first summer of being non-drinkers approached, our thoughts turned to holidays. Could we survive a week away without drinking? Would it ruin the whole holiday experience? Perhaps we should try something completely different?

We settled on the Camino, picking a route that took us from Bilbao to Santander along the coastal cliffs of northern Spain. Aodhan had done a different section years before, meeting people with life-affirming stories to tell and getting to see the world in a completely different way. He assured me that I'd love it.

Once the decision was made, we began breaking in our boots. We would be walking 120 kilometres over five days on our Camino, so we needed to prepare. Once again, my weekends began to revolve around joy-making hikes, climbing through Glendalough Valley and soaring over the Guinness Lake in the Wicklow Mountains. Rounding the crest of a hill and surveying the landscape below that we had just carefully picked our way through. Sitting with a roll and a flask of coffee on a rock, black lake below, green mountains all around, birds soaring in the silence. A natural high better than any night out that I could remember.

The holiday was indeed different. Instead of lying by a pool or on a beach for seven days, we marched through fields and along cliff walks surveying the beaches below. When we got too hot, we would work our way down the paths into the coves below, stripping off and diving into the rolling waves. We stopped at towns and villages for lunches of outdoor tapas or hot chips at a busy beach shack, licking salty fingers and smiling at each other, delighted with ourselves. Icy cold bottles of Coca-Cola served with a straw instantly deleted any beer cravings.

Later on that week, however, Aodhan had an acute wobble in his alcohol-free journey, but those days hiking the dirt trails were a perfect first step into holidays without alcohol.

While my fitness improved, my sugar cravings went the opposite direction. The reason for this was two-fold. For one, my reward system that I had relied on for so long was gone, so I needed something to take its place. Instead of a bottle of beer at the end of a long week, I would substitute chocolate. My addiction to Green & Black's may have kept them in business that first year. Instead of deciding between a Rioja or a Chianti, I would choose between Maya Gold or Butterscotch, or perhaps the 70% dark, or on particularly weak days, sickly sweet bars of white chocolate. It was my Friday night reward, my Saturday night treat, my midweek bump.

I also learned that it wasn't just my mental substitute

– my body was in fact missing the actual sugar that it was used to receiving through alcohol. It's recommended that women ingest no more than six teaspoons of sugar a day, but alcohol is laced with it. Drinking a six pack of cider (4.5%) over the course of the week will add a jaw-dropping 32 teaspoons of sugar to your intake. A bottle of white wine (12.5%) contains eight teaspoons of sugar. But the sugar craving is short term and far easier to break than the habitual craving for alcohol. Within a few months, I was back down to a manageable level again.

What I find interesting is how when it comes to sugar, calories and weight gain, we will look at absolutely everything we possibly can before we look at alcohol. I know people who have gone vegetarian, done seven-day juice fasts, joined eye-wateringly expensive gyms, cut out dairy, won't eat after 6 p.m., obsessively count calories, measure ingredients and generally obsess over their stomach and dress size, yet will not enter into discussions over cutting out alcohol.

After my first 100 days alcohol free, I checked my I'm Done Drinking app, which recorded my numbers. I had saved myself 30,000 wasted calories. To put that into perspective, a 10k run burns off about 600. That's a hell of a lot of running.

So why is it such a no-go area? If someone really wants to drop a dress size but isn't willing to give up alcohol in order to do it, what does that mean? That they are drink dependent? Addicted maybe? An alcoholic?

It's an uncomfortable thought and one that I, like many others, had pushed away in the past. Why are you asking me difficult questions? Shut up and stop ruining my buzz. It's social suicide not to drink. I'll just cut down. I'll drink spritzers. Or slimline tonic. I'll substitute my drinks for less food …

It's not just the empty calories either. It's the takeaway on the way home, the greasy breakfast in the morning, the midday sugar snack and Lucozade to keep you going, the day spent on the sofa, the carb-loaded dinner to comfort you to sleep. When you swap all that for endless energy and healthy living, for many people the excess weight that they struggled to lose for years simply falls away unnoticed.

But there are factors far more serious than weight gain to consider when it comes to alcohol.

I grew up in the 1970s and 80s, when smoking was a rite of passage. The Marlboro Man hung from billboards and Matt Dillon, the coolest of cool actors at the time, always had a cigarette hanging from his lips. The top decks of buses were a hazy teenage den and smoking in cinemas only added to the atmosphere. As we hit our teenage years, packets of smokes would begin to appear in the pockets of our 501s or rolled into the boys' T-shirt sleeves à la Marlon Brando and James Dean. With scrawny arms and freckled Irish skin, The Wild One they were not. Still, smoking was cool and forbidden and nothing was going to tell us otherwise.

My friend Samantha owned a car at 17, unheard of in 1990s Ireland. It was a black and wine Citroen 2CV that sometimes needed to run off a Doc Martens shoelace as an accelerator cable, but it was everything to us. We would stick our favourite Technotronic tape in the deck, roll down the windows and ride around town thinking we were the business. Smoking only added to our unshakeable belief that we. were. the. shit.

I was a late adopter of smoking within the group. Almost everyone except myself and Jenny had started at about 16. Now that we were frequenting pubs every weekend, I found myself bumming more and more cigarettes. I was that annoying friend that 'didn't smoke' and therefore didn't need to buy them. Until I did.

By the age of 19 I was just at the stage of buying the odd packet of 10 Silk Cut Purple on a Friday to see me through the weekend when my dad, with the sixth sense of a reformed smoker, cut in with an offer that I couldn't refuse. If I agreed not to smoke for the next year he would give me £250 right then and a further £250 at the end of the first year. I took his offer, didn't touch a cigarette again and let him off the second payment as a thank you for saving me from a vice that I realised I didn't need.

Over the years since then, smoking has become less and less socially acceptable. The dangers became clearly evident to our brains from the gruesome images that appeared on the packaging. It certainly helped make it less attractive an option for me (along with my dad's cash, of course).

But when it comes to alcohol, no such warnings have ever been in place. No notices that might make us think twice about knocking back a naggin of vodka in a field or a bottle of Brunello in a fancy restaurant. In fact, alcohol labels are becoming even more glamorous, with special edition bottles of gin and arty designs on cans of craft beers.

I've always known that smoking causes cancer. But did you know that drinking alcohol causes cancer? I certainly didn't. How many cigarettes are in a bottle of wine? The researchers of a 2018 study say that drinking a bottle of wine a week carries the same lifetime cancer risk as smoking up to 10 cigarettes a week in women and five in men.

Drinking alcohol increases the risk of mouth, upper throat, oesophageal, voice box, breast, bowel and liver cancer. Of the cancers linked to alcohol, drinking causes more cases of breast cancer than any other type in the UK. Breast cancer is the most common of the alcohol-related cancer types.

But that's not all. Smoking and drinking together is like supercharging both drugs in their cancer-causing abilities. Cigarette smoke contains over 70 cancer-causing chemicals and alcohol makes it easier for these harmful chemicals to enter the cell lining in the mouth, throat, larynx (voice box) and oesophagus, which greatly increases the risk of cancer developing in these areas. The cancer-causing chemicals of smoking piggyback onto your drink and into your body. It makes total and terrifying sense, but it's not something most of us will ever have thought about.

What I do know is that now that we are waking up to that knowledge, there are a lot of angry people about. People who have lost loved ones to cancer possibly caused by alcohol. People who have cancer themselves possibly because of alcohol. Would they have made different choices had they known the facts? Perhaps. It would have been nice to have had the option. Why were we kept in the dark until now?

I came face to face with this reality when I was training for the marathon. One perfectly normal morning as I was rushing to get out of the house to go to work, I went to the bathroom and saw blood in the toilet. I said nothing, thinking it was a once-off that would go away on its own. But a couple of weeks later it happened again, worse than before. So I did that thing that you know you shouldn't do but that everybody does. I Googled it. Immediately one of the options on offer for my self-diagnosis was colon cancer, so that's what my brain latched onto. At work, on long runs and late at night lying in bed in the dark, the fear of cancer would pop its ugly head into my thoughts. Worst case scenarios flashed through my head. I eventually spoke to Aodhan about it and decided to go to the doctor, for peace of mind if nothing else. It worked – the doctor said to monitor it and see if it happened again. If it did, I was to go back to him.

It helped relieve the worry and I went back to normal.

Until a couple of weeks later. I was on my way back home on a 13-mile run and knew I would need to stop for a toilet break. Fortunately there was a public toilet nearby, so I ran in, pausing my all-important timing app, with the aim of making it the shortest pitstop possible. But when I sat down, an explosion of bright red blood filled the sides of the bowl. I stared at it in shock and panic. Something was seriously wrong. I ran back out of there on shaky legs that had nothing to do with the distance of my run.

I went back to the doctor, worried now. He sat at the other side of the desk, worried too.

'I'd like to get you in for an urgent colonoscopy,' he said. He talked about how it could be nothing, but it was best to be straight – it could be cancer, so we needed to find out.

Urgent and *cancer* were the only words I could recall from the conversation.

I sat in my car outside my house for a long time. The kids were inside and I wasn't ready to pass through into that reality yet. I rang Aodhan, hands shaking, voice quivering. He said all the right things, placating me, making me feel better. But I could tell he was worried too.

I imagined the worst possible thing I could think of: my children losing their mother. This could not be happening. And yet it happens every day to hundreds of people all around us.

I took a deep breath, got out of the car and went into the house.

'Where have you been?' my daughter Kaya asked.

'I just had to pop to the doctor,' I said, hoping that would be it.

'Everything okay?'

'Yes, fine. I just might need to go for some tests,' I half-lied.

'Are you sure you're okay?' she asked again with concern. Teenagers seldom take an interest in their parents' health.

Maybe it was because I very rarely go to the doctor. Maybe it was because I carried with me an air of shock and disbelief. Maybe she saw something hidden under the mask on my face. I'm not sure she believed my assurances.

I told my sisters and was met by complete denial. 'No. Of course there's nothing wrong with you. Of course you don't have cancer.'

'You can't,' said Siobhan. 'You're the healthiest person I know. You're running a marathon and you don't drink, for fuck's sake.'

We agreed that if I had cancer, it was wholly unde-served and the world is not a fair place. As if everyone who did have cancer had somehow brought it upon themselves, which of course I knew was not the case. Cancer can strike indiscriminately.

I spent the next two weeks in a hazy 'what if' state, pulling the kids in for long unwanted hugs and drifting off in numbed daydreams.

When the day of the colonoscopy came, which iron-ically was the day after the marathon, I was frightened but ready, thankful that I would soon know one way or another. Aodhan drove me into the hospital and sat with me until they came to collect me. I wondered what it would be like to have to face it alone.

They gave me a robe and a bed and I waited, curtains drawn, an old man and a middle-aged lady on either side. 'I didn't like it at all,' the lady whimpered to the nurse as my heartbeat quickened.

Eventually they wheeled me into the small waiting area beside the theatre. Bright strip lighting and alien machines and screens bore down on me. It wasn't until the sedation had been given and trickled through my blood-stream that I could relax.

Later, in my drugged-up state, the doctor told me that everything looked good and the full results would be sent out. I shouldn't worry.

I wasn't sure if I had imagined the entire conversation, so it was only when the results did arrive that I stopped worrying. I was fine. With my marathon completed, the issue disappeared and I returned to normal life. It was all probably caused by the gruelling training sessions.

I am acutely aware that many, many people do not get the results they prayed for on tests such as these. Lives are turned upside down, emotions are ripped through, futures are agonised over. The world is indeed not fair.

But there are high percentages of some cancers that can be attributed to or increased by alcohol. That's not to say that these cancers are self-inflicted, but that if we knew what caused them, we could make better choices. We know that smoking causes lung cancer, so we choose not to smoke. If we all knew that drinking causes breast cancer, would we choose not to drink?

The Irish Cancer Society's (ICS) website has a section called 'Alcohol and Cancer'. It states:

> Alcohol is a known cause of cancers of the mouth, throat (pharynx), voice box (larynx), oesophagus (food pipe), breast, liver, bowel ... You can reduce your chance of getting cancer if you avoid alcohol or only drink a little. Even a small amount of alcohol can increase your risk of cancer. It's not just people who have a 'drinking problem' who are affected. The more you drink, the higher your risk.

While we all know that drinking affects your liver, how many of us know that it's a cause of breast cancer? The ICS goes on:

> Even small amounts of alcohol can increase the risk of breast cancer. A recent review of evidence showed that even one standard drink a day could increase the risk of breast cancer by 5 per cent. And the risk increases the more a woman drinks.

Alcohol is now classified as a group 1 carcinogen by the International Agency for Research on Cancer (IARC) as there is a proven, causal link between alcohol and several types of cancer. There's simply no denying it or hiding from it any more.

But alcohol doesn't just cause cancer. According to the World Health Organization (WHO), the harmful use of alcohol is a causal factor in more than 200 disease and injury conditions.

Knowledge is power. It may lead to uncomfortable feelings and difficult decisions, but it's better than having crucial facts hidden from us. So now that you know, what are you going to do with that knowledge? Perhaps we can all take out the chequebook and try to bribe our children with it.

Chapter 6

Friendships and
Sober Socialising

'Oh my God, are you not over that yet?'

My sisters weren't happy. Why was I being so boring?

I found that one of the hardest things to deal with in the early days was other people's reactions. And I get it. As a drinker I never, ever trusted anyone who didn't drink. 'Ugh! Why would they do that? What's wrong with them?' It also made me uncomfortable when there was a non-drinker in our midst on a night out. Were they judging me? Was I slurring? They're too sensible, too judgy, too sober. Here, let me shift seats, I have to get away from this person who is on another planet from me right now.

And now I am that person, ruining people's fun just by my sober presence. I get it.

For the first 30 days, I mostly hid myself away from social occasions. I didn't have the confidence to go out to the pub or for dinner with friends without a drink in hand. The more I thought about it, the crazier I realised that was. I didn't feel comfortable talking to my friends without a drink. Why was that? I knew that if we were all sitting in a coffee shop drinking americanos and eating cake, I would be fine. I knew that if we were at the playground with our kids, I would be fine. But in a drinking environment when I wasn't drinking? Not fine.

But I couldn't figure out why. Was it because of the pressure to be 'fun'? Was it because having a drink in those situations was ingrained in my blueprint? Was it because I was worried that they were worried that I was judging them?

Four years down the line, I'm still not sure but I think I have the answer. Since I was about 17, I had been drinking socially. Every meal out, every pub visit, every night on the town. Hundreds and hundreds of social engagements over 30 years that all involved alcohol. My association between socialising and alcohol was deeply entrenched. Every one of those days or nights out fed into who I was when I was 'out'. I didn't know how to be just Katie in a social situation. I didn't know who I was in those places without a drink in my hand. I would have to learn to be this new person, the real version of me. And that was terrifying, because I didn't know if I liked her.

My social awkwardness probably began when I was about 16 and pubs and nightclubs entered my world. I was always quiet but had a close group of friends I felt entirely comfortable with, so I could be wholly myself. But as wider groups started to form and the usual teenage experimentation began, I found myself feeling shy and uncomfortable more and more often. I would sit silent and listening as far more gregarious and confident friends entertained the circle. I felt like I had nothing to offer that anyone would want to hear. I was quiet. I was boring. Who even was I?

Hold on, though, look what we have here! A magical liquid that takes all that away! It makes you feel confident and comfortable. It disposes of your inhibitions. It allows you to become the best version of you so that other people can see it too. And it takes away that uncomfortable awkwardness. It makes you feel like you belong.

And so you begin to drink. Every weekend gathering, every pub visit, every party, every night out. You know who you are now. You know this 'social' version of you. It's fun and exciting and you get to be the person you want to be.

Years pass. Maybe even 30. And you can't imagine the person in the pub without a drink in hand any more because you never got to know her.

While my first 30 days had involved hibernating most weekends, I knew that I couldn't do that forever or I would become a crazy cat lady, holed up with a bag of knitting and no friends. To be honest, that didn't even seem like a bad solution. I like knitting. And cats.

Other than that fancy dress Halloween party in the woods, I had managed only one other night out in that first month. Even though it was with good friends in the local pub, that, too, had felt awkward and uncomfortable.

I had whispered my order to the barman and smuggled it back to the table, hoping that no one would notice the non-alcoholic Erdinger in the sea of gin and tonics. 'Why are you off the booze, Katie?' they asked immediately. I didn't even have a good answer, not one that I could snappily reply with. There were so many little things, not one big reason. I wasn't an alcoholic. I wasn't pregnant. I wasn't going through a crisis. I wasn't sick. I wasn't on a detox health buzz. I was just aware that there might be a better life waiting for me outside of alcohol. A niggling doubt that maybe it had been holding me back, that there was a better version of me available.

So I explained that I was just doing it to support Aodhan, but I'd be back on the booze in no time. I was mostly silent for the rest of the night, shifting in my seat, far too aware of myself.

I wondered whether I just needed more practice, maybe in a safe space. So I organised a Sunday lunch with some friends and family. Just a small group I felt comfortable with. Plus Aodhan would be there, so I'd have a sober companion.

It was lovely. And I didn't really miss the wine at all. I was full of energy and hosting like a pro, topping up glasses and clearing away dishes. But then the meal was finished and so was I. The drinkers, however, were not. They sat for hours more, as I would have in the past, contentedly drinking through that warm glow of full stomachs and red wine while I wiped another counter clean and waited for them to call it a day. They left at about 7 p.m. – a perfectly respectable hour – but I was exhausted. Turns out that I'm not able to while away five hours at a dinner table without alcohol. I wrestle with the conundrum of whether this is a good or a bad thing. So maybe home entertaining wasn't the right way to go yet either. Maybe we needed to go back to the pub.

The next night out was with Aodhan's friends. Again, awkward. I overthought everything. Were they wishing I wasn't there? Were we ruining their fun? Should I tell that story? Was I being too quiet? Was it time to leave yet?

Funnily enough, I realised that at no time was I judging anyone else. The new non-drinker in your midst isn't counting your drinks and rolling their eyes at your slurred speech and repeated story. They're too busy thinking about themselves.

Although I thought I was failing at each attempt as I navigated this new social life, the truth is that I was actually relearning how to be me. I was discovering how to be social without alcohol.

Next to be ticked off the social calendar list was a gig, indelibly linked with a few drinks to loosen up and enjoy ourselves. It was 29 November 2016 and we are almost at the two-month mark of being off alcohol. This one was surprisingly easy.

I'm not sure how I discovered Hinds, an all-girl Spanish garage band just out of school, but I'm glad I did. And I clearly wasn't the only one. The downstairs of The Academy in Dublin was nicely buzzing with hip young things and older musos. I'd like to think we fall somewhere between the two, but nursing our sparkling waters, we were definitely outliers. The barman had practically snorted at me when I had asked if they had any non-alcoholic beers. So that's a no then. It was either Coke from a gun (not as exciting as it sounds) or a Ballygowan. We shifted around uncomfortably, skirting the edges of the room.

But as soon as the support band took to the stage, everything changed. A prowling mess of young men in lacy crop tops and tweed jackets, they unexpectedly blew us away. A little bit Ramones, a lot unique. They were new on the scene and they were called The Fontaines. We'd never heard of them and neither had anyone else in the crowd. When they finished their set, the charismatic lead singer came over and hugged the woman standing beside us. It was his mum.

The girls from Hinds took up the mantle and the room returned to a throbbing, joyous party. I'd been to many, many gigs before, but none of them sober. This time, I was fully aware and taking it all in, my senses heightened. I wasn't constantly running to the bar or the loo during the set. I was enjoying myself. Without alcohol. It was a major step forward. After the gig we jumped into the car and drove home, an added pleasure in itself. No walking through freezing streets, no depressing Dart or expensive taxi rounding off the night. It makes going out so much easier – we just needed to get used to the being out part.

A couple of weeks later, early in December and two months after our last drink, Aodhan and I headed to Dingle for Other Voices, a music festival that takes place in tiny venues across the village. Crowds are crammed into churches, halls and pubs. Big names mix with up-and-coming artists and the whole town comes alive with twinkly fairy lights and excited smiles. Guinness flows freely, pints upon pints lined up on long wooden bars. It's a step back in time with a foot in the future. And the entire experience is indelibly woven with drink.

After a four-hour drive over mountains and fields, we finally arrived and headed into the village to get our bearings and stretch our legs. The west coast of Ireland is incredibly beautiful – striking rocks jutting out from crashing waves, cold winds racing over ancient ruins. We entered the village and passed pubs that had been unchanged for decades, each one like a warm hug, welcoming you with a pint in one hand and a whiskey in the other. I wondered whether we could do this.

The first place we went into was an American tourist's dream, a pub-cum-hardware shop where hammers and nails are for sale alongside beers and spirits. We sat up on the high stools at the bar and I discreetly asked whether they had any alcohol-free beers even as my head was telling me to take the weekend off and order a pint of goddamn Guinness, for fuck's sake.

The barman laughed. Good joke. And then saw that we were serious. He got flustered and I could see his thoughts passing across his face. Shit, she's an alcoholic. Can't drink. Quick, say something.

That's the thing about not drinking – everyone thinks there's a tragic backstory. I should probably invent one.

Amazingly, the poor barman recovered himself and found a couple of non-alcoholic Erdingers. After the first cold sip I realised that we would be okay. We were part of the festival experience going on all around us. We're there, in it.

Later we wandered across the road to Paul Geaney's bar and found an unknown band setting up. But hold on, I recognised those crop tops – it was The Fontaines again. They played a raucous, sprawling set right up in our faces before marching off into the night. Within a couple of years they were the darlings of the Irish music scene, headlining festivals, running sell-out tours and releasing critically acclaimed chart-topping albums. Those two chanced-upon gigs, when I was totally sober, were pretty special. We knew we were seeing something remarkable and we could fully take in (and remember) all of it. In my drinking days I would probably have been more interested in where my next drink was coming from, and who cares about the support act anyway.

The next few days passed in a jam-packed whirlwind of new bands, traditional folk, famous faces, talks, food, long walks and happiness.

Enjoying Other Voices without alcohol was incredibly easy. We quickly discovered that we didn't need the pint of beer in front of us to have alcohol in it to make the weekend great – it's perfect as it is. Perhaps even better.

It was another first ticked off the list and I felt myself becoming stronger. A sober Christmas didn't seem quite so impossible any more and we mentally signed up for the full 90 days, something that would have felt completely and utterly inconceivable just eight weeks before.

I've always loved Christmas. As a little girl I would count down the days remaining on the calendar, waiting for the body-bursting excitement of Christmas Eve. I would lie in bed that night trying desperately to fall asleep. I knew the rules. One fateful year I heard the bells of the reindeer outside and went from wide-eyed fear to knocked out cold in 60 seconds – it must have been the magic dust Santa cast over me. The excitement of finding the pillowcase stuffed full of gifts at the end of the bed the next morning. Running into brothers' and sisters' rooms at 6 a.m. – 'Look what I got! Look what I got!' – as plastic animals and fancy soaps spilled forth onto beds.

As the years passed and we all grew up, the excitement would revolve around the magic of the local pub on Christmas Eve. The pulling back of the heavy doors to the Burnaby, the whoosh of warm air from inside, then the ear-bursting blast of a hundred conversations. Families and friends returned home from every corner of the world, all converged into one bar. So much to catch up on, so many remembered faces. The 'Welcome homes' and 'So good to see yous' echoing all around. It would take a good 10 minutes of inching through the crowd to get to the bar and then you would be lost to the night. I would tiptoe into the house after closing time, eat the Crunchie from my selection box that Santa still left on my bed, and fall into a deep sleep.

We had a long-standing family tradition of 7:30 a.m. mass on Christmas morning, but what made sense with four excited kids no longer did with four hungover young adults. Instead, we managed to drag ourselves to the 11 a.m. sitting. Afterwards, duty done, we would light the fire, pop open the first of many bottles of champagne, put out the smoked salmon and begin to settle in for the day. Bubbles and presents were followed by Christmas dinner with bottles and bottles of good red wine. We could sit for five, six, seven hours at the kitchen table, ploughing through countless bottles before moving on to port, brandy, whiskey and then often back to wine. There would be singing and fiddle playing and storytelling and bantering and I loved it. And then we would retire to the living room to play the annual board game. By now my mother would rightly be delighted with herself for pulling it all off for another year and could finally relax. She would sit in our midst, crying laughing from her efforts at the game of Pictionary that she clearly didn't understand.

We followed the same routine for 20 years and even now we still need a democratic vote, complete with side whispers and brown envelopes, to change any of the traditions. So the year Mum suggested that we all go to mass on Christmas Eve instead of Christmas Day so that she would have more time for dinner prep the next day left us all reeling. How could she?! Until we realised that it also gave us more time in the morning to recover from the night before, so we 'reluctantly' conceded.

The next day, we would rise with the banging heads of a two-day hangover – which had been led in by weeks of pre-Christmas events – and we would start again. As the years went by, we swapped houses to my brother and sister-in-law's for St Stephen's Day celebrations. Ever the perfect hosts, they would meet us at the door with gin and tonics and put on a smorgasbord of delights for us all. We would happily graze for the rest of the day while performing our blind wine-tasting competition. This involved each of us bringing a bottle of carefully selected red wine, which would then be covered up and poured into glasses to be rated by us, the obvious connoisseurs. We took great pleasure in outdoing each other with our choices of €30 bottles of Barolo and carefully selected Bordeaux. We all thought we were sommelier experts, but each year the cheapest Rioja came out on top. It makes you wonder.

In fact, actual sommelier experts are often 'fooled' by cheap wines too. Study after study shows supposed 'experts' being fooled by trickery such as dyeing a white wine red (they couldn't tell) or decanting the same wine into different bottles (they couldn't tell).

So is that €30 bottle of wine really that much better than the €10 one? The truth is that if you poured the cheap wine into the expensive bottle, most of us wouldn't even notice the difference. A whole industry has been built around the intricacies of flavour, but mostly you either just like it or you don't. So much has to do with setting, expectations, memories and emotions.

But that first Christmas, there was no denying that it would be very different. Challenging in a new way. If I wasn't drinking and Aodhan wasn't drinking and Liam wasn't drinking, then the whole dynamic had changed.

'Exactly,' my sisters huffed.

The run-up to the season was different too. Instead of a calendar full of drinking engagements that broke my body as well as my bank balance, I now carefully chose the ones I wanted to go to. Dinner with the girls, a meet-up with old school friends and my work Christmas party were all on the list that first year. It's the last one that frightened me.

When the evening arrived, we rocked up in our sparkly dresses and glittery make-up. I dressed the part if nothing else. A fire twirler and (very randomly) a didgeridoo player had been employed to welcome us at the steps outside the venue, so it's clear from the off that the evening would certainly not be boring. Chefs had been brought in to prepare wild and foraged food and the stairway was adorned with fairy lights and garlands. I was nervous and unsure of myself until we were seated in our pre-arranged places. I'd been placed beside Aisling, a young fashion editor who is both cool and glowing. I felt old and boring.

And then she mentioned the unmentionable. Was I not drinking? I launched into a complex explanation of One Year No Beer, my ex, my brother, Aodhan's health and the kitchen sink. I'm sure I saw her sparkly eyes glaze over.

'I don't drink either,' she said with a flick of her long blonde hair. As if it's the most normal thing in the world. 'I don't really like it.'

And that was that. I made a mental note to myself to be more Aisling in future and we got on with the evening.

But later, when the tables were pulled away and the DJ arrived, the worst of my fears was realised. There was dancing. Everyone was dancing. It was too early to leave and there was literally no escape, so I closed my eyes and threw myself reluctantly into the music. Surprisingly, it wasn't as bad as I had feared. My first sober dancing experience was ticked off the list.

The rest of the run-up to Christmas and the day itself were similarly insightful. I didn't feel overwhelmed by my ever-growing to-do lists – for once, I was organised. Presents had been purchased without expensive last-minute panic buys and I was full of energy and feeling good.

On Christmas morning I was as excited as the kids, fully present in their presents. I didn't feel the sluggish haze of the bubbles from the night before or the frazzled anxiety waiting to be calmed by a Buck's Fizz top-up. Instead, I was well rested and ready to go. We followed the same traditions as always, but it felt totally different. The champagne with the family was replaced by non-alcoholic beers and fake gins, and honestly I hardly minded. It was a calmer sort of chaos as wrapping paper was ripped off and hugs dispensed. I felt happy and grateful as I looked around, taking it all in. Dinner was a more muted affair than normal, and over the course of the day I took regular 'peace breaks' to recharge, disappearing to a quiet room or for a walk along the seafront. For an introvert, socialising without alcohol, even with your own family, can deplete your resources. Plus I was still learning this new way of life. I enjoyed it, though. There was a quiet satisfaction to the day. It felt better this way. And as if to prove it to myself, the next morning I went for a run, passing a few similarly smug individuals on the roads at 8 a.m.

I have a new and completely untested theory on why some people hate Christmas. While for many it's a combination of factors, from tragic childhoods to unrealised dreams of their future, for many others there's no particular reason, just a dread in the pit of their stomach and a desire for it all to be over. Could it be that alcohol is the root cause? So many nights out over such a short period of time leaves our minds and bodies exhausted. I've been there many times, dragging myself out for another session when all I really want is my PJs, fluffy slippers and a curry in front of the TV. We go because we feel obliged to, because we don't want to let anyone down, because we said we would, because he might be there, because we don't want to miss out. But it drains us and we end up paying the price eventually.

So does our wallet. We beg and we borrow to spend money we don't have on drinks we don't want until we wake up in January hating booze, hating our lives, hating ourselves and hating Christmas.

And then we forget about it all for another year until it starts approaching again, and we feel the anxiety rising in our chest as our entire being recalls the despair from 12 months ago.

With my first Christmas ticked off my list, I headed into the new year. New Year's Eve, always a despised occasion of fake revelry, was slayed with a blissful night at home. And just like that, our 90-day alcohol-free challenge was complete.

So now what? We'd started with 30 days, moved to two months, then to 90 days. Neither I nor Aodhan were ready to return to drinking. Should we keep limping along month by month? Or bite the bullet and mentally sign up to the full 365 – a whole year without drink? What had seemed unthinkable before now seemed doable. In fact, the alternative – going back on the booze – didn't seem inviting at all. A year would mean ticking off many more firsts: weddings, birthdays, festivals, holidays. But with sober dancing accomplished, I was ready for anything. We dove in to see what happened.

The first wedding we faced was a big affair in a beautiful house in magical grounds in the country. I felt surprisingly at ease, a quiet confidence growing in me. I managed to sit at the table and enjoy myself. I wasn't nervously fidgeting or wondering what everyone made of us. I didn't care as much any more.

Nevertheless, at some point the conversation turned to the fact that we were no longer drinking, as it did every single time we went out. Friends, family, strangers – they just can't get their head around it. You're not an alcoholic but you *chose* to give up alcohol? Can't compute. They stare in wide-eyed wonder or shake their heads as if trying to remove whatever block is stopping their understanding. Nope. Don't get it.

But later in the night, they'll come back and admit that they would love to try it, they just know they wouldn't be able to do it. They want to know what it's like, how we manage, how hard it is, whether there's some secret we can share.

The fact that this happens so regularly that I've come to expect it reinforces my belief that there are many, many people out there stuck in negative relationships with alcohol. Why else are they so keen to break free?

For most, it's a complex love–hate affair. We love the initial endorphins that it brings, along with the associations we've come to expect from it – belonging, inclusion, safety, memories, bonding – but we hate the way it makes us feel afterwards – hungover, anxious, sick, ashamed, lethargic, embarrassed. We make promises to ourselves of 'no drinking midweek' or 'no drinking alone' or 'no drinking whiskey' or 'not more than two glasses or one bottle or, or, or…'.

But it never lasts. If you've ever made a promise to yourself like that (and really, who hasn't?), then chances are you don't really love alcohol and it certainly doesn't love you. So many of us are stuck in a dependent relationship with it, one that feels so normal because everyone else around us is in the same type of relationship. But suddenly, when faced with someone who ditched alcohol (hello!) and found a much more nourishing relationship, people begin to wonder – is there another way? Could I be happier without it?

What I found from my nights out sober socialising is that lots of people might not be ready to admit their interest in ditching the booze until they are boozed up – and then the truth comes spilling out. There's a deep irony in there somewhere.

Later on that night at the wedding, we both faced the dance floor. The lights were low and the music was good. It was as good a time as any to jump in, but we skirted around the edges watching for too long.

'Okay, I'm ready,' Aodhan said, and we're in. We didn't stop until it was time to leave.

As the months went by, we ticked off all the other major social milestones. We became more confident in our non-drinking social selves. We were learning a new skill, and that takes practice. Lots of it. The fact that we've been so hardwired to believe that alcohol equals pleasure means that it takes time to undo and rewire that belief. It's only through building up experiences without alcohol that we can do it.

A full three years after giving up the drink, we decided to take on the festival circuit. We bought tickets for All Together Now, the new kid on the block hit sensation from the year before. Smaller and friendlier than many of the other festivals, it's billed as a true music lovers' festival. What's not to love?

Quite a bit, as it turns out, but mostly before we actually arrived. We left as early as we could on the Friday to head down on the two-hour drive south for the weekend. Unfortunately, over 20,000 other people were also on their way and the back country roads were not ready for us. We spent five hours in barely moving tailbacks. The locals were the heroes of the hour. Rather than rolling their eyes and giving out, they appeared with shortcut directions, bottles of water and even toilet breaks in their own homes. We veered off left at the strong suggestion of one local man, but got caught head-on at the top of the hill with a tractor coming the other way. Aodhan pulled into a wooded area and a strange stench overpowered us. We were stuck. There was a long, loud and pained squealing coming from one side. An unearthly horror cry. Realisation dawned.

'Oh my God, it's a fucking abattoir.' I was in my worst nightmare and there was no way out. We rolled up the windows and I sat rocking in the front seat, sweat pouring down my face, anxiety rising. 'Oh my god, oh my god, oh my god.'

After what seemed like a decade of *Twilight Zone* horror, we escaped. This was not a good omen and not a good start to our first sober festival experience. I wondered whether we should have stayed at home instead. But as soon as we (finally) arrived at the site, all was forgiven.

We moved through the security line quickly. All around us the other festival goers were carrying heavy slabs of cans that they would drink warm over the next three days. Bags were being searched and questions asked. We had nothing to declare.

The blessedly short walk down the hill brought us to the first sleeping area, where colourful wooden pods lined the field like little fairy houses. We set up camp and headed into the festival area. Food trucks and bars lined the sides and we searched out suitable drink offerings. Alcohol-free beers were available, so that was us sorted for the weekend. We leisurely mooched around the site, getting our bearings. Like any other festival, there was an array of great acts we wanted to see over the weekend. What usually happens on these occasions is that you get to see one or two of the 'must-sees' on your list and then the drink takes over and you find yourself sitting on the grass chatting to random strangers and missing the music. This time, it was all about the bands. Friday night we went back to the start of our sober journey and watched The Fontaines (now Fontaines D.C.) finally take their crown as they headlined the main stage. Then it was on to the brilliant King Kong Company and a DJ set from Nenah Cherry. We headed back to our sleeping bags, tired and happy.

But it was Saturday morning when the magic hit. We woke up refreshed (when does that ever happen at a festival?) and joined the line by the campsite food trucks for coffee and pastries. Tired bodies, messy heads and mascara-ed faces surrounded us. You could see the suffering in their eyes. We got our supplies and practically skipped into the park. It was quiet and beautiful. The morning light breezed in through the trees as the stallholders began setting up. We chatted to a few, getting tips and information for the day ahead. We drank peppermint tea on the grass and found reggae brunches and ska dance-offs. We went to talks in billowing white tents and then stumbled on our highlight of the festival, an intimate and unexpected audience with Patti Smith. Two new fans were born.

Sunday was more of the same, with the evening spent running between stages to see much-loved and hard-to-choose-between acts – John Grant, The Good, The Bad & The Queen, and The National. It was the best time I'd ever had at a festival and I was sober. I couldn't believe it myself.

No missed music, no lost friends, no drunken decisions, no soul-crushing hangovers in a field and lots of extra delights I hadn't expected. As we packed up bright and early Monday morning to escape the three-hour tailback on the way out, we agreed that this was the way forward. We booked the next year's tickets as soon as they went up.

I've heard of many people not feeling able to ditch the drink or going back to it after a break because of the loss of social connection. It's certainly understandable.

'What if my friends don't want to hang around me any more?' one asks. I wonder whether I should tell her to find new friends. If alcohol is the only thing binding you together, I'm pretty sure there are better friendships out there waiting for you.

I'm very fortunate to have good friends who quickly accepted the new me. One has even begun the awakening herself. Lisa texts me randomly and I love being brought back to the newness of stepping out of the fog.

> *'Daily waves of contentment and excitement rolling through me!'*

> *'Overwhelming feeling of all that hasn't been achieved and so much time having been wasted.'*

> *'Mind is literally blown.'*

> *'So happy walking around the house all morning thinking of things I'd like to do today. Who am I?!'*

'Day 18 musings. I feel like I am on holiday from myself. I think 30 days is too short – finishing after a month would be so easy to fall back into your usual self. Think after 90+ days the old life will be less familiar. Sounds ridiculous – will develop thoughts here!'

'Is this real life?'

Chapter 7

Children and Parenting

It's a sunny day in July and the boys are at a playdate in a friend's house for the afternoon. Aodhan and I are in our first year together, still drinking and still escaping from real life at every opportunity. The kids will be staying with their dad that night, so we head into Dublin for the day to make the most of our little slice of freedom. We plan on market browsing and pub crawling.

We stroll around the side streets of the city, dropping into bookshops, art galleries, music stores and indie pop-ups. Interspersed with this are stops for cider in the sunshine at Trinity's Pavilion and a Guinness in the darkness of Anseo before hitting my favourite, The Palace Bar. There's nothing like a traditional Irish bar on a Saturday afternoon. There's a secret handshake feel to it, like you're the only ones in the world in on the story. All members playing for the same team, escaping the world for a while.

As Aodhan goes to the bar to order a second pint for us, I check my phone. Six missed calls. My veins freeze. Something is wrong. I check the call log – Kristian, my mother and the mother of the boys' friend have all tried phoning over the past hour. Something is *very* wrong. I curse myself for not being there for them and my need to break free. Selfish! Why did I do that? Why wasn't I home with them? I step outside the bar and with shaking fingers dial Kristian's number.

'Where are you?' he demands before I have a chance to speak.

I am standing in a side street in Dublin with shoppers and drinkers passing by, all oblivious to the disaster that is unfolding at the other end of the line. I can't breathe.

'Baxter had an accident.'

I close my eyes. The world stops.

'He's okay now. We're on our way home from the hospital.'

I listen to the rest of the tale with a deep exhale. He had fallen on broken steel and the gash in his leg ran deep. His friend's mum had tried to get hold of us, first calling me, then my mother, then Kristian. They'd taken him to the local chemist first, who had told them stitches were needed. Kristian had already had a drink that day and I was unavailable. My sister's partner had saved the day, driving them to the hospital.

Later they showed me graphic pictures. White calf muscle showing through red flesh. He still has a scar today, a reminder of the day I went off duty.

The guilt was crippling.

It's a strange thing, the guilt. It's not like parents aren't allowed to take time off from their children, but when you do and something bad happens, it's hard to escape the feeling that you failed them. That you should have been there for them. But you weren't.

One of the things that struck me after that day was the fact that four phone calls had to be made on that sunny Saturday afternoon to find a driver. Saturday afternoon pints were clearly on the table for more people than just me. Because that's what we do, isn't it? Sunny weekends spent at barbeques or in beer gardens, the kids running in and out with bags of crisps and glasses of Coke. One of our locals has a bouncy castle on the grass outside where parents can pay for the privilege of having their kids entertained while they enjoy a few scoops. It seems ingenious. Happy kids, happy parents, happy hour (or three). But is it really? When both parents are drinking, who does the emergency run in the middle of the day or night? I don't know, but maybe that's one of the reasons why our ambulance services are so stretched. And what are we teaching our kids about pub culture? Look at us all having so much fun because of alcohol!

I spent many an afternoon in that pub, kids rushing in with sweaty heads and smiles looking for another fiver so that they could have more time on the bouncy castle. Fantastic. I got a well-earned break and they had a few fun-filled hours. I have no doubt that the associations being made in their young heads were far from healthy.

When I was seven years old, my father had his fiftieth birthday party in our garden. All his friends and neighbours were invited and each of the kids got to have a couple of close friends over too. There was drink, food, music and big steel barrels of fire. It was the most exciting thing that had ever happened to us. There was a bar outside, which consisted of big plastic drums filled with water and ice housing endless beers. In the kitchen there were boxes of terrible wine, with plastic taps that you pressed the tops of to dispense cheap red and white offerings. My brothers, aged just nine and eleven, along with their friends crouched under the taps and poured it straight into each other's mouths when no one was looking. It felt illicit and exciting to my young mind.

We grew up with clear lessons around alcohol. Don't drink. Be careful. Alcohol is dangerous. But what we saw all around us was very different. Drinking is fun. Drinking is sophisticated. Drinking is cool. And so we fall into step and follow, only to perpetuate the whole cycle again for our own kids. Don't drink. Drink is bad. Oh, look at me! This is so much fun! Is it any wonder that our relationship with alcohol is complicated?

I used to laugh along with the rest of the internet about wine o'clock and 'mummy's juice'.

The most expensive part of having kids is all the wine you have to drink.

Yep! I would think.

To reduce stress, I do yoga. Just kidding. I drink wine in my yoga pants.

When they start to whine, I start to wine.

When my three children were all under five, I wrote an article for a paper titled 'I'm not a desperate housewife, but

I like my glass of wine'. I wrote about the stress and boredom of being a stay-at-home mum to three young children and feeling the need to ceremoniously acknowledge some adult time at the end of another long day. Myself and Kristian would share a bottle of wine most nights, and a poll of friends had showed that many did the same. We had all come to rely on the crutch and the ritual. Inevitably the next day we would feel a little more tired, a little less enthused about the 10 hours that lay ahead of us. By the time 7 p.m. rolled around, we would be gasping for something to take the edge off and make us feel better. Alcohol was making motherhood harder rather than easier and I didn't even notice. Soon after exploring our drinking habits for that piece, we managed to break the cycle of the daily bottle. It was tough that first week, but after that it seemed crazy that we had been sinking six to seven bottles a week between us.

The weekends, though, remained sacrosanct. Friday night wasn't Friday night without a celebratory drink in hand. But as the kids hit their tweens and teens, their own social lives began to take off. They would be invited to friends' houses after school for their own Friday celebrations, which would inevitably involve staying for pizza, ice cream and maybe a movie. 'Pick them up about 9 if you like!' the text would come through and my heart would sink. I'd silently curse mother and child for imposing a Friday night alcohol ban on me.

As soon as I went alcohol free, the potential emergency runs and weekend taxi service ceased to be an issue. I was available any time, day or night. Pick-up from a disco at midnight? No problem. Child feeling sick on a sleepover? I'll be right round. It made me feel more responsible as a parent and more in control of our lives. The slight anxiety that sat on my shoulders was gone, the what-ifs becoming so-whats.

The other major gain in the realm of parenting that I felt, almost from day one of giving up alcohol, was my energy levels. Looking after kids is exhausting, whatever their age. The baby years are physically breaking, what with the lack of sleep, the heavy lifting and the constant tailing of a tiny toddler with a death wish. And then there's the emotional side – retaining your patience during the twenty-sixth tantrum of the day on three hours' sleep, this one because he wanted his socks off and then his socks were off, the tortured screams echoing through the streets. The physical and mental exhaustion of parenting young children is second to nothing I have ever experienced. Adding alcohol to the mix means that your body and mind are desperately using any reserves they have left to process it, and that makes the days 10 times harder. Personally I found that as my kids got older, it became easier. Their relentless need for you diminishes. It becomes more about logistics, emotional support and of course the never-ending battle of breaking up fights with siblings.

But it is still draining. The calendar of events that need to be ticked off each week. The schoolwork that needs to be checked. The friendships that are wobbling. Who needs to be where and when? Who hasn't checked in today and when did they say they would be home? Hormones bounce off walls and onto trampolines. Sometimes they bounce into faces and all hell breaks loose. Splitting up the twelfth fight of the day is as trying as dealing with the tantrum-throwing toddler.

Parenting takes herculean reserves of patience plus endless energy. And drinking depletes both of those resources.

Once alcohol had been taken off the table, both literally and figuratively, it was apparent how much of an effect it had had on me. With my newfound energy came endless plans. We would go hiking or swimming or adventuring. I no longer talked about doing fun stuff with them on the weekend and then not see it through because I was too tired. I would commit to driving to the place to do the thing that Saturday because I knew that I would not be hungover. The most unexpected gain from giving up drink was how much easier it made the logistics of my parenting life. Lifts, planning and outings all fell into place and my messy mothering began to take a little more shape.

On one of the mornings that I decided to do a sunrise swim, one of the boys asked me to wake him up so that he could come too. I didn't believe that he would, but when I whispered in his ear he rolled out of bed and into the car. After our freezing alarm call, we sat on the beach together and watched the silky water turn liquid gold as fire coloured the sky. He rested his head on my shoulder. It was a moment of silent perfection and we carried it home like secret treasure in our chests.

There were other mornings when all three braved it, flasks of tea and Pikachu onesies at the ready. I'd like to believe that we were building both memories and a love of nature that will stay with them long after I am gone.

Just to be clear here, I still shout at my kids. I still lose my temper with them and then feel guilty. Giving up alcohol doesn't suddenly make you Mary Poppins (and anyway, who knows what her patience levels would have been like without magic on her side?). But it does give you the chance to be your best parenting self. It doesn't rob your family of fun memories. Being alcohol free gives your kids the best mum or dad you are capable of giving them with the resources you have available to you. It also gifts you unexpected pleasures that are so much deeper and purer than those at the bottom of a bottle.

In those early days of parenting, as the kids grew up, they watched us drinking almost every Friday and Saturday night. Some Sunday afternoons we would all go to the pub to meet friends or else join family at my mother's house for a home-cooked roast dinner. Both events inevitably revolved around alcohol.

Obviously watching us all week after week would have impacted my children's view on drinking. It's fun! It's grown up! Everyone does it! As children we observe what goes on around us and that becomes our truth. It's uncomfortable to think about, and when I was drinking I would have become dismissive of anyone who might dare to mention it. Articles on the damaging effects of alcohol were dismissed in favour of extremely debatable 'red wine is good for your heart' research, which of course we all lapped up and passed on because that was what we wanted to hear.

But when I stopped drinking, I became fascinated with a child's view on it. They hadn't been sucked into the machine yet. It wasn't a part of their daily lives. So what did they really think about it? I asked my own children and their cousins. 'Alcohol makes some grown-ups scary,' said one. 'They're like different people when they're drinking,' said another. 'They think they're funny, but they're not,' said a third.

Ouch.

One online forum comment I saw from a dad struck me and has stayed with me. He said that he was sitting at home at his desk one weekend and his 11-year-old boy brought him over a bottle of beer. It was his way of saying, 'Hey there, Dad, take a break, you're working too hard.'

At 11 years old he had already associated alcohol with relaxation. The implications of that one act woke the father up and he realised what he had been inadvertently teaching his son. Others have similar stories, something that shifted their perspective enough to let a chink of light in so that they could see things from their own child's perspective. Clare Pooley writes in *The Sober Diaries* about how one afternoon she accidentally sprayed beer over her two young kids. She tried to laugh it off and make a joke of it, but seeing her small innocent children covered in alcohol shifted something in her and she realised that things had to change.

'Remember when you used to bring beer up to bed, Mum?' one of my kids asked me recently. Now used to living with a non-drinking mum, he was aghast and amused that this had ever occurred.

I was outraged. I had never, ever gone to bed with a beer! As *if!*

'Yes you did,' he said simply.

But then I remembered what he remembered. It was Friday night and the kids had all been watching endlessly annoying YouTube videos in the sitting room. We have a small house, so I'd escaped to the only other room I could for a bit of peace and quiet – my bedroom. I sat on the bed reading my book and drinking a bottle of Peroni. At bedtime the kids all came upstairs into my room and we said our goodnights.

And there it was. In his head, I used to go to bed with a bottle of beer, even though I probably only did that a handful of times in total.

But now I don't drink. Neither does my brother. Neither does my partner. Neither did their dad for an extended period of time. Big family occasions are a slightly quieter affair. Weekends are still fun. My children are learning that they don't need alcohol to live a full and complete life. I'm not totally blind, of course. I know they will experiment. I know they will have to take their own path and find their own way. I know that it won't be long before I am checking their eyes and seeing if they can walk in a straight line when they come in late at night. But I'd like to think that I've now shown them that there *is* another path. That there is an alternative. Going by my own experience, I don't think many people growing up in Ireland actually realise that.

My oldest child is now 16, the age that I started drinking. My sisters, by the way, think this is hilarious – the fact that I was so old. They were creating dolly mixtures from our parents' drinks cabinet as soon as they hit their teens. My older sister was pulled out of a local over-18s nightclub at the age of 14 by our outraged father.

'Sorry, he's drunk again,' she lied over her shoulder at the bouncers so that she might be allowed back in again the following week. At 14 I was still saving my money for the best high top basketball boots I could afford and going out for pizza with friends was a huge thrill.

Getting my kids to the oldest age possible before they start experimenting is really my only hope. I know that they will succumb to the temptations – in our culture, it's virtually impossible not to. But more and more research is pointing to the fact that the earlier a person starts drinking, the more likely they are to become drink dependent in later years. Drinking before the age of 15 increases their dependency and affects their brain development.

'What do you think about me not drinking?' I asked my 14-year-old when he was trapped in the car with me – the only chance I get to have conversations bigger than where are you going and what time will you be back.

'I think it's really good,' he replied. When pressed, he said it was because I got to spend more time with the family and it's better for me and my health. I'm not sure if he was just reciting what he thought I wanted to hear, but at least it made him consider it.

'And do you think you'll drink?' I asked.

'Maybe when I'm 18,' he paused. 'Until I'm 20 and then I might stop.'

Ah, the innocence of youth. If only it were that easy.

To be honest, if he made it to 18 I'd be thrilled, but I know his peers will begin their experimentations before long and I can't really imagine him standing on the sidelines.

How do we stop this culture of underage drinking? I don't have the answer to this. But role modelling a different way as well as having open conversations and education about the risks have to be part of it.

I told him about the latest research and how the younger you start, the worse the effects. He nodded his head wisely. But then I told him if he was ever in trouble to call me, that I wouldn't be cross, that his safety is the absolute most important thing.

I can't help but wonder whether he considers that this is, in fact, me telling him that it's okay to drink after all. Navigating the fine line between warning them away from alcohol and being there for them when mistakes are made is a balancing act I haven't quite mastered yet.

When I was a teen, many of the worst offenders among my peers were the ones with the strictest parents. They let loose with abandon and often faced the consequences. Myself and my best friends, Jenny and Mo, came in family positions way down the pecking order (fourth, fifth and seventh children, respectively). Our parents had been there, seen that and practically given up by the time it came to us. By the age of 16 we were allowed to go to the nightclubs and the parties on the beach. We were given the freedom we needed, so we had nothing to rebel against. So while we took part in the teenage experiments, we never railed against the world or went off the rails. As the years progressed I got as drunk and high as anyone else, but the entry was definitely delayed. Which I only now realise was so important.

Other parents took the 'it's better under our own roof' path, believing that giving their children and their friends a safe place to drink was the best way of keeping it under control. This turns out not to be the best option either. Professor Deirdre Murray, who is a consultant paediatrician at Cork University Hospital, states that there is strong evidence that the earlier you start drinking, the more likely you are to suffer from problem drinking in later life. Why? Because if we are drinking before we have had time to develop our personality and our social self, then we come to rely on alcohol as a crutch. But the brain itself is also affected. The adolescent brain is developing rapidly, especially the frontal lobe, which is responsible for decision-making and emotional response. When we pour alcohol into it, these functions are stunted, meaning our whole future person is changed.

Teenagers start drinking for a number of reasons – because they think it's fun, because their friends are doing it, because of outside influences such as media, marketing or watching their parents, to escape problems or to seem grown up. Usually it's not just one reason, it's a little bit of all of them.

We went through it all as teenagers ourselves, but how do we navigate it as parents? Drinkaware (which incidentally is funded predominantly by large drinks companies, just so you know…) has a handy map to follow. These are the cues:

P – Proactive

Be proactive in discussing alcohol with your children. Don't wait for an alcohol-related incident to occur. Having a conversation about alcohol early will help your child to understand alcohol and its effects. Ultimately, this will help them to develop a healthy attitude towards alcohol, giving them the best chance to make sensible choices about drinking in the future.

A – Activities

Encourage sports, hobbies and social activities that keep your child active, healthy and fulfilled. Boredom and having nothing to do is often stated as a reason why some teenagers start drinking. So why not help your child get involved in activities that are of interest to them?

R – Rules

Don't be afraid to set rules in relation to alcohol use. Children need boundaries. However, it's important that you clearly communicate your expectations about alcohol with your child and that they know and understand the consequences of breaking those rules. Discussing this openly encourages mutual respect and trust.

E – Example

The example set by parents with their own drinking affects a child's behaviours and attitudes towards alcohol use. It is useful to think about your own relationship with alcohol and what messages your drinking habits could be sending to your child. Remember, you are the most influential person in your child's life.

N – Notice

Take notice of what is going on in your child's life. Who are their friends? What are their interests? Where are they spending their free time? Parents have a critical role to play in knowing where their children are and who they are with. Getting to know other parents and guardians can also give you a better picture of what is going on in your child's life.

T – Talk

Talking matters because effective parenting cannot happen without it. Good communication is the key to building self-esteem and resilience in your child. Communication is a two-way process and accepting that teenagers may see things differently is the first step in discussing issues effectively with them. You may be surprised how much teenagers will confide in you if they feel you are really listening to them.

I've lost count of the number of times I've heard the continental method as a theory for parents to follow.

'In France, they give children diluted wine so that it teaches them about moderation in a controlled environment.'

'I much prefer to let them have a couple of drinks at home with their friends so that I know what they're doing.'

Unfortunately, all the research shows that, for Irish teens, parental supply of alcohol actually increases the risks. According to an article on RTÉ on why young people are drinking less than older people, it doubles the risks of bingeing and more than doubles the risk of harm. Those that are given drinks at home are *more*, not less, likely to drink more than their peers. Perhaps this works in continental countries that don't have the binge drinking culture of Ireland or the UK, but for us it doesn't.

In 2013, when our children were five, seven and nine, Kristian and I moved the family to Spain. It was a last-ditch effort to reinvigorate our lives and our relationship – although it was never said out loud to anyone or each other. We lasted only six months there, but it was long enough to notice the cultural differences, and the chasm between the drinking patterns of the young Spaniards versus the young Irish was all too evident. Spanish youngsters would congregate late at night in town squares, big groups of excited boys and girls out for the weekend. So far, so familiar. But as I watched, I noticed that they would sit with a single drink each in front of them for hours, chatting and laughing with each other. Sometimes they would leave to move on to another location, often not even another bar. The ice cream parlour across the street was a popular hot spot. At 17 and 18 years old, their weekends involved staying out until the early hours with only one or two alcoholic drinks. This is not the case for our teens.

It's no fun reading about the risks of alcohol to our kids, especially when we know there's not much that we can do to stop them from trying it. While the prevalence of smoking in 15–16-year-olds dropped from 41% in 1995 to 13% in 2015, and has a government target of 5% for all demographics by 2025, drinking has shown no such extreme drop. It's still the norm, and although rates are decreasing, most teens will drink during their formative years.

When I asked my now 16-year-old daughter how many people in her friend group smoke, she wrinkled her nose. 'I don't know anyone who smokes,' she said, clearly disgusted.

When I asked the same question about drinking, she looked out the car window and hummed along to the radio.

So do we stick our heads in the sand or shrug our shoulders and say that it's a rite of passage – or do we inform ourselves and try to steer them to a better path?

For me, the more I learn, the more I wish I could protect them from it. But I also know that coming down too strong could have the opposite effect. So I'll continue to throw out bits of information, hoping that some of it might stick while waiting for the world to catch up on seeing the crazy relationship that we have with alcohol. What I've found was that once I saw alcohol for what it really is, there was a moment where all I wanted to do was go around and shake everybody that I love and scream in their faces, 'This is madness! We are literally poisoning ourselves!' But instead, I sip my Diet Coke and watch the chaos unfold around me.

When I let myself think about the drinking years that lie ahead for my kids, I worry deeply about them getting into cars with drunk drivers, or walking home on dark roads and being the victim of a hit and run, or getting into dangerous fights, or being raped, or molested, or becoming pregnant, or suicidal, or having a tragic accident, or making a really bad decision that will stay with them for the rest of their lives. And honestly, I'm not even being over-dramatic. I know people that every one of those things happened to when I was growing up. They were somebody's sons and daughters.

Some decisions made through drink are foolish – but others are deadly.

Chapter 8

Unexpected Joys

It was the early days of going sober and I was getting my legs waxed in the salon. Myself and the beauty therapist chatted about what we were up to for the weekend and the conversation turned to drink. I apologetically explained that I was off it for a bit, so there wasn't much happening in my social sphere. She told me that she'd been off it for ages.

'Have you not discovered the joys of breakfast yet?' she asked, perfect eyebrows raised. I had not. 'I switched from dinners out to brunch dates a long time ago,' she explained. Interesting. So instead of faking it at raucous restaurant meals, breakfast dates with friends, family and partners are made instead.

Up to that point, weekend breakfasts had always been a hungover affair. Dark glasses and heavy head. Sipping orange juice and strong coffee with big hopes that the carbs and fat of the next course would magic away the pain. Of course, it never did.

I walked out of the salon with smooth legs and a plan. The next day, Aodhan and I went for a Sunday morning brunch date in our favourite café. Sweet crunchy waffles and fresh berry compote. We surveyed the other customers – shades on, slow movements, suffering evident. We smiled smugly at each other and turned another page of the Sunday papers.

Little joys like this were unexpected, and they were everywhere. From obscenely productive mornings to being a better parent, these were the things I hadn't factored into my experience at the start. However, I soon found that saving money, having better relationships, a clean(er) house, feeling all your emotions, getting better sleep and having more time all came as part of the package.

Mornings in general became an absolute joy, my most productive and happiest time of the day. In the first months of giving up alcohol I used my early morning energy to complete my Digital Marketing Diploma, then I used it to write my first book, then to train for my marathon. Mornings gifted me with beautiful sunrises and magic memories. And all before school runs and starting work. I have achieved more in the past four years than I did in the past 14. At the moment I'm rising again at 6:30 every morning to swim 500 metres in the sea before coming home to write while the kids are still sleeping. I'm not Superwoman, not by a long shot, but when I read back on those achievements, I can't help but be proud of them. Each one I took on as a major goal and chipped away at it until it had been accomplished. It's a huge life lesson I've taken from this whole experience. Figure out what you want. Chunk it down. Do it. Being alcohol free allows you not only to find the clarity to figure out what it is that you want, it allows you to do it too.

Aodhan and I took the kids to Wexford for a week one summer. We brought books and board games and notebooks and big plans. Holidays and weekends away have become more about what they should be and less about escaping, bottle in hand, only to come home from the holiday needing a holiday. Nowadays our escapes are retreats. They are about family and fun. They are about stopping to look at the bigger picture. Taking time to look at the present – where we are and where we want to be. Planning for our future instead of blindly sleepwalking into it.

I sat Aodhan down in the garden and gave him a pen, then started asking questions. What are your personal development goals? How long will it take you to achieve each of them? What are your financial goals? What do you need to do now? My sister had joined us for a few days and appeared just as we were finishing the exercise.

'Jesus Christ, what is she doing to you? You poor fucker,' she said.

'I know,' Aodhan replied, 'but weirdly, I'm actually enjoying it.'

But I know this works. My one-year goals were to run a marathon, write a book, buy a new car and start a pension. And I ticked them all off. My long-term goal is to buy a forever home. That one seems a bit more tricky to achieve, but I'll keep you posted.

We made time for fun on that holiday too, honest. We rented bikes and cycled round Hook Head. We hunted out secret beaches and spent hours in the lapping waters. We got chills down our spines in the most haunted house in Ireland and toasted marshmallows in fire pits. It was simple, old-fashioned time spent together and it reset and recharged each of us in its own special way.

My newfound productivity levels are, I believe, a mixture of clarity of mind and energy of body. Without alcohol in my system, my body is able to perform like it's meant to. My internal organs are no longer heaving under the heavy weight of processing the poison, so there is a lightness in me. And my head is clear. I'm bubbling with positivity. Who knew that life could be this way?

'I have done 100 days alcohol free, saved €1,000 and dropped a jean size' shouted the headline of the *Irish Independent* article I wrote after the first three months. My I'm Done Drinking app had calculated the figures after I put in my details on day one. A round of drinks in the pub or a bottle of wine in a restaurant (€30), a pack of beer for the fridge (€10) plus two bottles of wine (€30) came to €70 a week. It seemed like a lot of alcohol, and a lot of money, but I felt it was fairly accurate. Needless to say, not everyone thought my spending was 'normal'. '€10 a day and she says she's not an alcoholic? Yeah, right.' When you say it like that, I could see their point. But it's surprising how the money adds up.

Being totally honest, I knew that this would be a normal week for me – but I also knew that some weeks, if I had a night out I would stick €70 or more in my pocket before leaving the house and come home with nothing. While spending €10 a day on alcohol seems like you might be an alcoholic, spending €70 on a night out doesn't. Sometimes I would go out to dinner with friends and then on to the pub, so that was €30 on a restaurant bottle of wine, €30 in the pub on a round, then maybe €30 more on another one a little later. Actually, I wouldn't really remember where the money went. It just seemed to disappear through my fingers, like a bad magic trick. I would bring out as much as I could afford to spend that night and there would typically be nothing left when I checked my pockets the next morning. Or my card would take the hit and I wouldn't realise the damage until the end of the month when my empty account caught up with me. At the time, I considered it normal. But is it?

'How much would you spend on drink on a night out?' I asked some friends.

'About €100,' one said. 'Pre-dinner drinks, wine at the restaurant, pub after that…'

'I could spend €50 in the pub,' said another, 'then €20 in the off-licence on the way home.'

'€100, easy,' shot back another.

'Yep, sounds about right,' came a further response.

Aodhan's friends gave similar responses. It seemed like the agreed average. And that's without the taxis, fast food or anything else.

Now that I'm not spending any of this money on alcohol, I find it much easier to get through to the end of the month and my next pay day. I can justify buying that new dress or getting that family takeaway. I've also started to book in a regular massage so that every six weeks my back, neck and shoulders are pounded into a state of nirvana. I walk out floating on clouds. After a while, I decided that it was time to finally get my future in order. I started that pension. Better late than never, I told myself. At first it was a tiny figure, the most I could manage. Then as the years went by I started adding more to the monthly deposits. It's not huge, but it's something. Knowing that I am building for my future takes away some of the anxiety. (Note to any twenty- and thirty-somethings in the audience – don't cash in that pension, even if it seems like a great idea at the time/the only way/you'll never actually get old. It's not and you will. Dammit.)

As the meme goes, 'Did some financial planning and looks like I can retire at 65 and live comfortably for 11 minutes.'

Let's just say it's a work in progress.

'Are there any unexpected benefits to giving up drink that you didn't foresee?' I asked Aodhan.

He paused for a moment and then nodded. 'I think I'm a nicer person now.'

This was unexpected. I hadn't actually considered it before. And I wasn't sure that it was even true – he's always been a nice person. In fact, the mutual friend who introduced us in the first place had described him to me as being 'almost *too* nice'. He's one of life's good guys.

'How so?' I asked, not convinced.

'I have more time for people now. I consider them more and would go out of my way to help them, whereas I might not have bothered before. And I've more patience.' I thought about it for a moment. It *was* true. He was even more supportive of friends, family and others now.

I turned the beam on myself to consider how much nicer and more helpful I was those days. Sadly, it's still searching. I don't think I've changed in that regard (yet). I've made a mental note to myself to work on it.

One thing I do notice, though, is that I have more time for people I would previously have ignored or avoided, especially on a night out. At parties or nights on the town I would have gravitated to The Fun Ones – the drinkers, the laughers, the ones that sparkled. Anyone not drinking or too quiet or too boring would have been overlooked after a couple of glasses. But now I realise that they are often the most interesting ones. They are the ones with the deep thoughts and considered opinions. They are the ones that can still make meaningful conversation at midnight.

It could be someone's granny, some odd-looking misfit in the corner or the quiet girl in the crowd sipping her non-alcoholic beer and watching the world. We all have stories to tell and it's only by listening that you really uncover and discover people. I'm far more ready to listen these days.

The other surprising thing is the depth of sober bonding. While those deep-and-meaningfuls that you have when drunk are often in fact meaningless, the ones that happen when sober bring real connection. During my drinking days I'd become best friends with random strangers more times than is logical. I've also walked past people in the street, both of us deeply mortified, because the weekend before we'd thought we were soulmates and now realised that we barely knew each other, and certainly not enough for her to have shared that story that only her closest friends should know. Getting to those levels of sharing should take years of establishing a friendship built on trust and respect. Then it means something. Thinking you are at that level just because the gin told you so is always going to end in regret.

Work parties are a disaster when it comes to this. Usually devoid of deep friendships and with lots of alcohol, we often share more than is appropriate for the relationships we have. Many times in my twenties I slunk into work the next day, full of embarrassment at telling Yvonne from accounts what I really thought of her boyfriend or having listened to Susan sharing stories she really shouldn't have. So many conversations with inappropriate people at inappropriate times that in the cold light of day felt spine-shakingly wrong. Those conversations didn't lead to friendship (unsurprisingly), but if Yvonne's true friend had sat her down to explain why she was so much better than her cheating fella or Susan's best friend had listened to her story and then helped her find the support she needed, then those conversations would have been worthwhile, maybe even leading to healing and better choices.

There have been many nights that I've put the world to rights with strangers in a kitchen at 3 a.m. At the time we would think we were part of a renegade crew – same opinions, same views. My people. But the next day we would all wake up with that hollow feeling in our gut and only a vague recollection of each other.

Drunken bonding isn't real. Now when I have those kitchen conversations it's with people who I find genuinely interesting and it's usually on a beach or over a coffee. We share a story or a view for what it is and I come away feeling like I had a genuine moment.

* * *

My house has always been messy. I like to think it's because I'm creative, but more likely it's just that I'm lazy. Cleaning and tidying has never been top of my to-do list – in fact, it comes very close to last place. When the kids came along it got out of hand. 'What's the point?' I would ask myself. 'It will only get messed up again within an hour.' Besides, I was just too tired. So the house stayed messy.

As they grew up I tried to get on top of things, but I just never had that tidy gene. Even when I spent a whole morning cleaning, it never looked like it should. My daughter, Kaya, on the other hand has it in spades (definitely from her dad Kristian's side). She only has to walk into a room and replace a cushion and it looks like a stylised Instagram shot. Her bedroom regularly gets made over into a haven of perfection. I'm like the messy teenager around her.

'Mum, could you replace the top of the toothpaste when you use it, please?'

'Mum, can you please just wrap up the cheese when you're finished with it?'

'Who didn't clean their plates after breakfast? I tidied this all up last night!'

Hello, Saffy.

I wasn't quite *Ab Fab* status, but it wasn't too far off.

My siblings are all the same, so naturally we blame our mother. She in turn embarrasses us in public.

'She's a terrible slut,' she told her friends one day as they were sitting drinking coffee in her living room. She was talking about my sister, who lives beside her and happened to be sitting right there in the room too.

'Mum!' my sister shouted, appalled at the attack.

'What?' she said innocently. 'You *are* a slut. A domestic slut. Is there another meaning I've missed?' She looked around wide-eyed and innocent.

Apparently, the term *slut* used to mean a woman with low standards of cleanliness. So I guess we're a family of sluts. You learn something new every day.

Within weeks of giving up drink I had energy to burn, so I started to tackle all the household jobs I'd been putting on the long finger for years. My wardrobe got a big clear-out and a small update. The overflowing kitchen drawers got resorted. I repainted the kitchen from boring, bland Magnolia to a deep blue Denim Drift and my days were instantly transformed. I moved on to the sitting room, a fresh coat of light grey making everything feel calmer. Toy boxes and bookshelves were sorted and for once the house felt clean and orderly. My slut status washed down the drain with the dirty dishwater.

Four years later, my house still gets out of control more often than I would like. With three endlessly hungry children and no dishwasher, it's often a losing battle to stay on top of the kitchen, but I always have the energy to tackle new projects when I need to. I've realised the importance of the space we live in. How decluttering helps to free the mind and how a chaotic house breeds a bad mood. Although it may not come naturally to me, I'm getting better every day.

Just don't ask my daughter for her opinion on my levels of cleanliness though.

* * *

When I did my first triathlon, I had no idea what I was getting myself into. My brother Liam was one of those Lycra-clad obsessives who was always off cycling through the Wicklow Mountains or running 25k to Dublin to collect his race number for the next day's event.

'Do you think I could do a triathlon?' I asked him one morning over tea in our mum's kitchen. I had just done the 10k Women's Mini Marathon and reckoned I was pretty fit. A triathlon seemed almost impossible, but enticing all the same.

'Of course you could!' he replied enthusiastically. 'I'll do you up a little training plan.' The training plan involved a 'trial' triathlon in just three weeks' time. 'It will be good practice,' Liam assured me. And I believed him.

How I didn't realise that this 'trial' triathlon would in fact involve me doing an actual triathlon, I do not know. But because it was part of the plan he had drawn up, it seemed like just a step along the journey, not the end point.

So I began training. I borrowed a bike and started slowly cycling up hills. I kept running. I bought a wetsuit and self-consciously wriggled into it at the water's edge.

'We'll just swim across the cove and back,' Liam said to me one morning. That 'just' seemed misplaced to me. Across the cove was pretty far. And deep. And I had to make it back. 'You'll be grand!' he said, jumping in.

The cold water made me gasp and the depth made me anxious. I was breathing far too fast and my pan-icked strokes were making things worse. With many starts and stops to regain composure, I did indeed make it over and back. I hadn't enjoyed it, but I'd done it. I was pretty pleased with myself, but I knew I had a long way to go.

For the next swim, we met at the same place and I expected the same route.

'We'll just swim out to that yellow buoy over there, then go over and back across the cove again,' Liam announced.

Wait. What?

'What yellow buoy? THAT ONE?!' I pointed at the bright plastic buoy happily bobbing in the waves in the distance. Not a fucking chance.

'You'll be grand!' he said, diving in.

Panicked breaths, deep water, trying to catch up, yellow buoy, swim over, swim back, touch land.

I had done it.

'Not a bother to you,' he said.

I knew it wasn't true.

The next swim was further still. From the cove, we would swim back along the rocky shoreline to the next beach before returning to our starting point. Approximately 1 kilometre.

My confidence was building and the swim over was manageable. I kept my breathing calm and my strokes slow. I was learning how to do this. But on the way back my arms got tired and my body got cold. We were caught in a strong current and I didn't seem to be moving no matter how hard I pulled on the water. Deep sea on one side of me, jagged rocks on the other.

'I can't do it!' I shouted at Liam through the waves.

'Course you can!' he shouted back. 'You're fine.'

I took another few strokes to nowhere. No way out of the water. Panic building.

'Liam! I can't! I'm not getting anywhere. I can't do it.'

'You can. Just keep going a bit further and you'll be out the other side.'

Head down, gritted teeth. I had to push through. There was no other way.

And suddenly, the strokes got easier. I was flowing through the water again. The fear dissolved. I was almost home.

We got out of the water and with what was left of my strength, I punched him. 'Don't ever do that to me again!'

'What? You were grand. Not a bother to you.'

His unshakeable confidence in me was not mirrored by my own.

As the race day approached, my nerves were off the chart. The distances aren't huge – 750-metre swim, 20k cycle and 5k run – but it's the putting them all together, the transitioning from one leg to another, the wrangling out of your wetsuit at speed and not knowing where you're going on the cycle.

When Liam picked me up at 6 a.m. on the day of the triathlon, I wished that I had never got myself into this mess. We parked up, got the bikes out, picked up our swim hats and numbers and set up our stations. Then we waited around to listen to the briefings. I felt sick.

My wave was on later than his. He set off and I was alone in the crowd of wetsuited athletes. Everyone looked fitter, stronger and more capable than me. And then finally it was my turn. I stood on the pontoon, jumped into the Liffey, took a few deep breaths and was off.

The race was tough, but at the same time enjoyable. Once the swim was done, I relaxed into the rest of the course, cycling through Phoenix Park and then back to drop the bike and run with wooden legs through the last stage. I ran to the finish line exhausted but incredibly proud of myself. I had done something that just weeks before had seemed impossible. My fitness had increased, but unexpectedly, so had my confidence. When you accomplish something that had seemed out of your reach, it's an unbelievable boost to your own faith in yourself. You prove that niggling little voice in your head wrong. Actually, you *can* do it. You are strong. You are capable. You are more than you thought you were.

Whether it's doing a triathlon, running a marathon or doing a couch to 5k, overcoming a fitness challenge has a ripple effect on your whole self. But so do other challenges – a new job that you don't feel good enough for, learning how to drive or writing a book. Each new 'I can't do it' turns into an 'I did it' achievement and your belief in yourself grows.

This is exactly what happened when I gave up drinking. But instead of ripples, it came in waves. While I white knuckled it through my training – which consisted of nights out in pubs without my crutch and being home alone on a Saturday night with a mug of herbal tea – once I had put the hours in and flexed my non-drinking muscles, they got stronger. I began to relearn who I was as a person. No riding the buzz of a few drinks to feel comfortable among friends or acquaintances. No taking the edge off the day with a cold beer. No hiding in a bottle to deal with life's disappointments or fears. Everything had to be dealt with head on. And the more I did that, the more my confidence in myself grew.

It was just like Liam had said – not a bother to me.

✷ ✷ ✷

Dealing with emotions without a crutch is difficult sometimes. Sadly, there is no escaping pain, anxiety, grief, disappointment, guilt or stress in life. At some point we all have to face them. Thankfully, though, there are plenty of magical moments to counterbalance them. But whether it's the magical or the mundane, in our culture we usually punctuate each of them with a drink.

Births, deaths, marriages – all life's major moments come with a drink. When my father died 10 years ago, the whiskey bottle came out. He had passed away in the early hours of the morning with my sister and brother by his side. As I woke up and came down the stairs of my mother's house, Maria took my hand and whispered, 'He's gone.' We stared at each other, not knowing what to do or say next.

'Can we go for a walk?' I asked.

We walked around the seafront and through the town. It was early. Coffee shops were opening up and morning routines were beginning. In a typically surreal grief-stricken moment, I wondered how they could all be carrying on as if it was just a normal day. Did they not know my father had just died?

We returned home and moved through the day. By early evening the wine bottles were out, blurring raw emotions, bringing some relief. It didn't pack enough of a punch for me, though. The grief in the pit of my stomach gnawed relentlessly at my insides and the only thing that helped was the sharp sting of golden whiskey hitting my throat and warming my chest. I sat on the sofa surrounded by family, quietly gulping. My mother told me to be careful. I didn't want to be. I wanted oblivion.

The days passed in a haze of sorrow and gratitude that I can barely recall. In a way I now feel that I did my dad an injustice by blocking out that pain. Shouldn't I have fully felt all the emotions that his death brought? I think it would have shown me how much he meant to me, to really hold that hurt in my body and soul instead of hiding from it. Sometimes I feel like I didn't fully process the loss. I simply pushed it away, waiting until it either got smaller or I got stronger. Perhaps I'm still waiting.

Drink dulls the initial pain of grief, but it also dulls other emotions. When we have something to celebrate, we automatically pair the occasion with alcohol. A bottle of champagne, a night out with friends, a party. Alcohol and good news go hand in hand, just like alcohol and bad news. But what I've learned is that I actually enjoy those moments more now. When Aodhan's fortieth birthday rolled around, we planned a big night out. A local restaurant by the harbour was booked – festooned in fairy lights and balloons, it was the perfect venue. All his closest friends are there. They were celebrating not just his birthday, but also his second chapter in life. When his marriage broke up they were as devastated as he was – a seemingly perfect relationship between two of their friends had been torn to pieces overnight. This night, though, is a celebration of him turning bad news into good fortune, of resilience and finding happiness.

We brought bottles of alcohol-free prosecco for ourselves and clinked glasses with others. I could see him taking in the night, appreciating everything he has – close friends, wonderful family, us, community. He was perfectly content. It was an ideal moment from which to set off into the next 40 years.

Other emotions aren't so wonderful to have to feel fully. Parenting has many joys, but it certainly has its fair share of challenges too. One of the areas that I constantly feel I am failing at is being the mum I thought I would be (welcome to motherhood). I'm shouty, impatient and cross far too much of the time. I was sure that once I gave up alcohol I would become that version of Mary Poppins that I so wanted to be, sprinkling childhood magic wherever I went. But while some aspects became easier, the emotional side certainly didn't.

When our daughter was born and wouldn't sleep more than two hours at a time, I was exhausted, frustrated and hanging on by a very worn thread. One night, after many hours of her refusing to sleep, I remember punching the wall of my room in absolute rage at the despair I felt, rising hours later with bruised knuckles and a sense of fear and shame. No wonder so many of us drag ourselves through those days, counting down to bedtime when we can pour ourselves a large glass of something and collapse on the sofa for an hour of peace before we do it all again.

These days, when it all gets too much I usually go for a walk round the town, headphones in, cursing at them under my breath. In the past I've been known to go for a drive and shout until I'm hoarse. Other times I'll rage, say things I don't want to and then hide in my room while the power of the feelings fades from my body. I despair at the attitude they throw at me, then grit my teeth through the dreaded homework time. But a simple note that says 'I'm sorry, Mum' left on my pillow or a silent hug on the landing and I'm back to being lovestruck.

Being a mother is all about extremes. There are moments of heart-bursting love, when your chest physically hurts from having to contain all the feelings. Watching them sleep, their downy cheeks and full lips making you wonder how you ever got so lucky. Or when their small limbs curl around you, enveloping you, becoming you, and you breathe in their sweet softness. The whole world and everything you need in your arms. Or when their clear, bright eyes look into yours and you can see the love deep in the blue or the green or the brown of their soul. It's an unexplainable, world-affirming, this-is-the-meaning-of-life feeling. It goes deep into your bones and remains there forever. Your love for them becomes a physical part of you.

But they can be the most annoying little shits on earth too. They know exactly how to push your buttons and oh, boy, do they enjoy pushing them. As toddlers they are infuriating in their inexplicable desires. They want their socks on, but not on. They want their dinner on the yellow plate, but now it's touched the blue one, so not that dinner. They rage against you with red faces and clenched bodies for not letting them put their hand in the fire or drink the fabric softener or run into the road. There is no reasoning with them.

As they grow, their independence asserts itself. They often want to do things before they are ready to do them and a wall of wills builds. You cajole and bargain and explain and compromise like a world-class hostage negotiator. Every day. For years and years and years.

And then there is the sibling rivalry. The fighting, the shouting, 'he touched me', 'she said', 'he said'. The slaps and wrestling and punches and wails. I used to get so frustrated that I would sit on the stairs and pretend to cry so that they would stop their fighting. It was the only thing that would shock or guilt them into quitting.

Parenting is a rollercoaster of emotions with peaks of love and depths of rage you never thought possible. You race past pride and wonder and climb long stretches of guilt. Fear snakes into your brain no matter what justifications you throw at it.

You never really feel like you are enough. You never feel like you are fully in control. You never feel like your job is done. (Except that time when they all argued over what music to listen to in the car and finally agreed collectively on David Bowie.) Emotions in parenting are big and powerful from day one and they don't ever stop.

There's no hiding from the emotions of parenting any more with a glass of wine in the evening or a gin and tonic while making dinner. I have to feel them. All of them. I feel that rage. I feel that guilt. I Google long articles on how to deal with a disrespectful child, how to teach mindfulness to kids or how to not lose my shit. I go for a run to release the pressure or head out for a walk to process the day. I make a plan and try to follow it through for more than a day. I don't pour myself a large glass of wine to relax any more. I don't hide. And I don't beat myself up the next day. It's not perfect, but it's real.

✳ ✳ ✳

I never had trouble sleeping – until the kids came along, that is. Given the chance I would go to bed early, rise early and get a good nine hours' sleep in. But babies have other plans. They don't like Mum getting, oh, I don't know, more than two hours in a row? Over the years I forgot what a full night's sleep felt like. I got used to operating with whatever their breast-feeding, bed-hopping, asthma-breathing bodies allowed. I got through my days in a daze, early morning coffees tag-teaming me through the first leg and then the thought of a glass of wine in the evening getting me to the next one.

What I didn't know at the time (and would I have cared even if I did?) is that alcohol disrupts our circadian rhythms, leading to tiredness, irritability, fatigue and confusion. Tick, tick, tick and tick. I once found myself driving to work on a road I didn't recognise – my concentration had left me midway through the journey and I had autopiloted onto a different route. I blamed the baby brain. Another time I lost my wallet. I searched everywhere in a panic before finally admitting defeat and phoning the bank to cancel my cards. When I went to make myself a cup of tea to commiserate, there was the wallet in the fridge beside the milk.

I was definitely not getting my required sleep at that time and I was suffering the consequences. 'But drinking helps me go to sleep!' I hear a lot of people say. And it's true. It does. In fact, it's one of the most relied-upon sleep aids there is. But the actual truth is that while it may help us to drop off initially, the rest of our night's sleep is negatively impacted.

There are two principal stages of sleep that we cycle through – REM (rapid-eye-movement) sleep and non-REM sleep – and these repeat throughout the night every 90 minutes or so. The balance of REM to non-REM sleep changes as you move through the night, so in the first half of the night the majority of those 90-minute cycles is composed of deep non-REM sleep, and in the second half the balance shifts to more REM sleep. The Sleep Foundation states:

> *Experts believe that this [non-REM/deep sleep] stage is critical to restorative sleep, allowing for bodily recovery and growth. It may also bolster the immune system and other key bodily processes. Even though brain activity is reduced, there is evidence that deep sleep contributes to insightful thinking, creativity, and memory. We spend the most time in deep sleep during the first half of the night.*

Falling quickly into a sedated alcohol-induced sleep means that we miss out on much of that crucial stage.

As the night goes on and our bodies process the alcohol in our system, we enter a lighter sleep with more frequent wakings instead of the natural regenerative sleep cycles. Add in trips to the bathroom, night sweats and snoring (all enhanced by alcohol) and it's no wonder our sleep isn't what it should be. Which, of course, leads us to wake up feeling like we haven't slept enough, then off we go again through another tough day.

This process happens to a greater or lesser extent whether we're drinking one glass of wine or one bottle. So even though my reliance on alcohol eased up as my kids grew older and began to sleep more, I continued to wake up tired. After 10 years of disturbed sleep, I hardly knew any different.

It didn't take long for the sweet, deep sleep of my clean body to hit me. I began to wake up rested, refreshed and ready for the day. I felt like sleep had done the job it was meant to do. A feeling I had long forgotten. Better sleep leads to more energy, more productivity, better mood, better metabolism, increased immunity and a general sense that life is good. And who doesn't want all that?

When we sleep, our bodies are busy processing everything we've done to it that day – flushing out toxins, repairing damaged tissues, regenerating cells and restoring energy. Sleep allows us to heal, recover and become our optimum selves. No wonder it has become a modern-day obsession.

Matthew Walker, a neuroscientist who directs the sleep lab at Berkeley, has spent more than two decades studying how sleep impacts health and disease. His book *Why We Sleep* became a bestseller, with fans such as Bill Gates. The entire book breaks down why sleep is so important and how to make sure you are getting enough of it. In it, he states that, contrary to popular belief, alcohol is not a sleep aid, and while it might help induce sleep, 'alcohol is one of the most powerful suppressors of REM sleep … Alcohol is a sedative, and sedation is not sleep.' Noted, Mr Walker.

One unexpected joy wasn't entirely unexpected. In addition to sleeping better, giving up alcohol also makes you live longer.

'Who cares!' say all the drinkers. 'I'd rather enjoy my life now and die at 75 instead of 80!' Which makes sense. If that was how it happened, but (sorry) it's not. One soberista called it 'a slow death', explaining that from your late forties on we are severely impacting the ability of our brain and organs to function for the next three to four decades. So it's not the case that we are living our amazing lives up to age 75 and then dropping dead, chopping off the last years of life with a guillotine. No, our body is slowly limping to the finish line, breaking down piece by piece along the way.

It seems dramatic, but since giving up alcohol it makes total yet unexpected sense. Smug though it sounds, I've never felt healthier. I now feel like I'm nourishing my body to give it the very best chance of staying in top form for as long as possible. Our bodies are incredible, intricate machines and we need to look after them, not abuse them. They're essentially all we have, our greatest and most precious commodity.

I'll take those extra five years, thank you very much. And I'll also take the run-up to them in the best condition I could hope for.

* * *

One thing I didn't factor into the alcohol equation is the time we waste, from whole days or nights in the pub to evenings at home with a bottle of wine and hangovers that rob us of next days and whole weekends. Aodhan reminded me recently that he often used to book an annual leave day off work purely in preparation for the recovery he knew would be needed following a heavy session, so a Saturday wedding or a golf weekend away would automatically have a Monday annual leave day attached. We now shake our heads in disbelief at the waste of it.

The gift of time is unexpected and wonderful. Life takes on a less frantic pace. I'm more organised than I have ever been. I have time to get out and enjoy myself as well as ticking off the things on my to-do lists and making sure my hectic family schedule is under control.

I also don't waste hours of precious time at events I don't want to be at. So many nights in the past I had drunk my way to enjoyment when all I really wanted to do was go home and get into my pyjamas. I remember sitting in pubs many, many times before closing, full to the brim of beer and trying to think of something that I could have that wouldn't fill me up and would allow me to keep drinking. 'What will I have? What will I have?' I would think, drumming my fingers on the bar. Sometimes it was a whiskey, sometimes a gin. Always the better answer would have been to just go home.

'Nothing good ever happens after 2 a.m.,' a friend would tut the next day with a sad shake of her head, having stayed out until sunrise.

Going out for a night at 7 p.m. and staying out until 1 a.m. means spending six hours drinking. Factor in the next day's hangover from, say, 8 a.m. to 2 p.m. (and sometimes all day), that's another six hours. So in total that's 12 hours out of 24 taken up by drink, with seven hours of bad sleep thrown into the mix. It doesn't leave much of a weekend. No wonder I felt like time was slipping through my fingers.

These days, my marker is midnight. Four hours of catching up with friends followed by a great night's sleep, an early morning swim and a whole day stretching ahead. I'd much rather have those life-affirming, highly productive extra few hours the next morning than using the last hours of the night having conversations I can't remember, then doubling up the wasted hours with a hangover the next day.

But by far the most unexpected joy and the real surprise of giving up alcohol has been that it didn't strip my life of anything. In fact, it's been the opposite. I thought I would be giving up, losing out, missing life, but actually life has become more fun, more exciting, more everything. There are the big accomplishments – writing books, running a marathon, ticking off my major life goals – but more importantly, there are the countless small joys every day that make it the best gift I have ever given myself. Sipping coffee in the garden after an early morning swim, taking my daughter out for lunch, wrestling with the boys on the trampoline, strolling hand in hand with Aodhan on a Saturday evening, mountain hikes, deeper relationships, a good night's sleep. Having the time, energy and awareness to do all these things is the gift that keeps on giving. These unexpected joys feel like the keys to a life well lived. And really, isn't that what we are all searching for?

Chapter 9

Challenges

My Day One of giving up alcohol took place mostly at the airport. We were leaving Amsterdam with sore heads and aching bodies. When I spotted those huge leather massage chairs across the room while we waited for our flight, the sight was akin to seeing a lifebuoy when you're not sure you're going to be strong enough to stay afloat on your own. I sank into its cushioned arms and spent the next 30 minutes getting pummelled into oblivion.

The first 24 hours after drinking is when your body eliminates the alcohol from your system. It's usually calculated at one unit per hour, so if you drink five pints that's approximately 5 x 3 units = 15 hours until the alcohol has left your system. One bottle of wine at 10 units is 10 hours. So if you go to bed at midnight, by 10 a.m. the drink should be out of your system (paid for with a bad night's sleep). That's the theory, anyway. My hangovers told a very different story. Sometimes I'd feel bad for a whole morning after a single glass of wine.

Flying into Dublin that day, I had zero desire to drink for the foreseeable future. But sure, who hasn't uttered the words 'never again' at some point in their lives?

On Day Two I had to get through a big day at work. Adrenaline got me to the end of the day, then the exhaustion hit. I later read that the mood-enhancing chemical dopamine that our brains produce is still depleted at this stage and our body is still fighting hard to replace all the missing minerals and glycogen that the alcohol nuked out of us. For anyone who drinks at the weekend, this is called Monday.

The next couple of days I was grumpy, sluggish and my sleep was broken. By Thursday I should have been having an 'almost the weekend!' loosener, but without it available or even on the horizon, I felt flat and a little low. What was the point of not drinking if I felt worse, not better?

This is the very first hurdle that causes so many falls. You have a big weekend because you know it will be your last for a while, then you feel worse than ever during the week so that by the time the weekend rolls around again you just want a little bit of joy back. So you throw your previously made promises out the window and decide you can't be bothered continuing.

We were on our first sober holiday together when the first real wobble happened, nine months after giving up. We had hiked 120 kilometres over five days as part of our Camino and we were finishing up the trip in Santander. Five days of walking over mountains, fields and beaches had brought us back to city life, full of bars, restaurants and tapas, spoiled for choice with incredible food and fantastic wines. We found a small tapas place a little off the beaten track, up a quiet cobbled street. We ducked under the low stone doorway and found ourselves in a candlelit cave-like room. The waiters were flamboyant and funny and the dishes circulating from the kitchen looked and smelled better than anything I'd encountered so far. The other diners were all Spanish, talking loudly and eating hungrily. It felt like being in the beating heart of Spain herself. As I looked around, I realised that it wasn't quite a cave, it was a cellar, and the walls were lined with bottles and bottles of incredible-looking wines. Labels of different years and colours peeked out at me, some covered in dust from the last decade, others newly placed and shining temptingly. Gulp.

We sat down and ordered from the extensive menu. Our tapas arrived along with our Cokes. We bit into the charred Padrón peppers, licking fat flakes of salt from our fingertips, and dipped slices of oily bread into rich tomato sauces. It was perfection ... except that I couldn't shake the feeling that it would be better with a thick, oaky glass of Rioja to wash it all down with.

'I'm going to have a glass of wine,' I announced to Aodhan impulsively, waiting to see what his reaction would be. I wasn't sure whether I was or I wasn't, but I wanted to gauge his reaction before I fully decided.

His head shot up, excited at first, then a vague disappointment crossed his face. 'Are you really?' he asked. 'You can if you want.'

I could see the thoughts flying through his head as his eyes flicked left and right and his mind began a what-if journey.

'I mean, we're on holiday?' I half-stated and half-asked. 'We could just have one glass with the meal and then leave it at that ...'

But my mind had already gone to whether one glass would be enough. Maybe one bottle? But that seemed like too much. I realised that if we did have a drink, be it a glass or a bottle, our run of 270 or so days would be over and we'd have to start again. And I really did want to get to the full 365 days.

Just like that, I had come full circle and had talked myself out of it. The moment had passed. 'Never mind!' I said to Aodhan as I picked up my fork and got on with the feast. 'I'm grand now!'

Aodhan, however, wasn't.

Although we finished the beautiful meal without talking any more about it, I had thrown him off centre. The little voice in his own brain had begun to go down the 'sure, just one drink won't hurt' route. We left the cellar and walked down to sit on the steps of the local square, which was, of course, surrounded by bars.

Aodhan wanted a beer. It was a deep, dark want.

He sat beside me very quietly as he silently wrestled with himself. To-ing and fro-ing, pro-ing and con-ing. I waited with him, hoping that he'd reach the same conclusion I had just moments earlier. Eventually one of us suggested getting an alcohol-free beer while he made his decision. As soon as he returned with the AF bottles, he was fine again. Back on track. I could physically feel the mood lifting. We were both relieved and grateful that he hadn't succumbed. He was on a thoughtful high for the rest of the evening. He had fought his first real battle with the demon and he had won.

One of the challenges anyone who gives up drink faces is the finality of their decision – and the temptation that brings. The thought that you may never drink again brings a feeling of loss. You're grieving the best part of what you've stepped away from. 'I'll never have a crazy night out/dance on tables/taste good red wine/live a wild life ever again.'

And so your mind begins to ask 'what if'. What if you only drank one glass of wine when you went out for dinner? What if you only drank once a month? What if you only drank on special occasions? What if you only drank on holiday?

The voices inside my head would get louder from time to time, drowning each other out. If life was feeling flat, I would wonder what rules I could apply that would mean I could bring back a little bit of the sparkle. But in truth, I knew it was a slippery slope. One glass becomes two, one Saturday night becomes every weekend, and before you know it you're back to square one. During these times I would find that a lot of my mental energy would be spent weighing it all up. Could I? Should I? Will I? Won't I?

I Googled 'drinking in moderation' and looked for answers in alcohol-free Facebook groups. The jury was out. It felt like it was the Holy Grail that people were searching for, but there seemed to be very, very few who made it there.

And then I read a quote by Harvard Business School professor Clayton Christensen, who said, 'It's easier to hold your principles 100 per cent of the time than it is to hold them 98 per cent of the time.' He called it the 100 Per Cent Rule and I realised that this was my answer. There was no point spending my energy going back and forth about whether to drink or not drink on every night out for the rest of my life. I would just commit to being a non-drinker and that was that. Decision made. Headspace free again.

Michael Jordan also followed this rule. He said, 'Once I made a decision, I never thought about it again.' And that's the key. Make the decision, commit and get on with your life.

Once the penny had well and truly dropped for me, everything became easier. My confidence in my decision grew, my motivation for continuing got stronger, my new identity became much clearer and the future me became more certain.

Reading other people's stories online and talking to those who tried to go back to a moderation path, it seems clear that unless you've always been a 'take it or leave it' kind of drinker, then drinking in moderation is far more difficult than not drinking at all. A study from the University of Gothenburg in Sweden backs this up. They found that those who want to drink in moderation are less likely to achieve their goal than those who set a goal of quitting drinking entirely. Of those they studied, 90%

of the people who chose total abstinence were still sober two years later, whereas only 50% of those who focused on controlled consumption succeeded in controlling their drinking. Which one was I?

'What was your biggest challenge to giving up?' I asked Aodhan.

'Finding out who I was without alcohol,' he said after a very short pause.

Aodhan had grown up in a busy, loving home with six siblings who brought him connections all over town. He was a popular kid, good looking and unfairly talented at every sport he took his hand to. But football was his main love and skill. He played from a young age and for multiple teams.

Like me, Aodhan was naturally quiet. His drinking career started very early and progressed quickly. He had a strong friendship group and, like so many Irish teens, their social lives revolved around drinking. The football teams he played for were packed with athletes full of bravado and testosterone. He drank to fit in, to feel at ease with himself. And then he just kept drinking. His drinking habits were no more and no less than others in his social and sporting circles, or indeed mine. Which meant that they were significant.

Like me, Aodhan didn't know himself without alcohol. He had to find out who he actually was. That learning curve was steep at first, and often uncomfortable. Having those awkward conversations, standing up to the pressure, second-guessing yourself, letting go of who you thought you were, easing into who you actually are, accepting yourself. It's a bumpy but fascinating journey.

But we were lucky. Having each other to lean on in those early days made all the difference. After almost a year off the drink, Kristian was struggling. He felt bored and stuck. He had tried weekend activities that didn't revolve around the pub, even joining a hiking club, but he felt removed from any real social connection. He decided that he would like to be able to go to the pub for a pint with a mate. He felt that he needed it. I was disappointed for him because I thought his mental health was better without it, but I understood. It was a difficult choice for him: the need for a simple social connection that helped his mental state balanced against taking a drug that worsened it. It was a classic catch-22.

For me, sober socialising was one of the biggest challenges. Getting to know who I was in a social situation without alcohol as a crutch could have undone me. Sitting awkwardly at the edge of the table, feeling very much on the outskirts of everything, was a tough task. For someone who is quiet at the best of times, I felt like I needed that loosener, that social lubricant that helped me feel like part of the crowd. Every new social experience brought nerves, doubt and then a renewed confidence – in myself, in who I am and in what I was trying to do. It's like a muscle that needs flexing and building.

The first pub trip, the first party, the first Christmas, the first bad news, the first wedding, the first holiday – they were all big steps up the mountain that felt tough at the time, but brought me to the incredible view from the top.

But the greatest challenge for me by far was other people's perceptions. At first I didn't feel strong enough to take on social situations without a drink in my hand. But little by little, at each new social occasion I slowly built up a bit of confidence. Unfortunately, though, as my confidence grew the opportunities began to dry up. Nights out occurred without me and I felt like I was an unwanted noose around the neck of partygoers.

I wasn't the only one. One night soon after we had started our break from alcohol, Aodhan was unusually quiet.

'Are you okay?' I asked him as we were going to bed.

'The lads all went to the pub tonight.'

I could see him wrestling with not wanting to be bothered by it and being bothered by it.

'Do you think they didn't invite you on purpose?' I said, voicing his thoughts.

'I don't know. Maybe?'

We talked ourselves round in circles until I just told him to ask them about it. Tell them that even though he's not drinking, he'd still like to be included. When he did, they were surprised. They had thought he wouldn't want to go. After all, what was the point of going to the pub when you're not drinking?

'Do they not realise I go out to see *them*, not just so that I can have a beer?' he asked me.

I decided that I would need to make this clear in my own circles too. Just because I wasn't drinking didn't mean I didn't want to go out. Perhaps our initial hermitage in the first few weeks had set the precedent, but whatever it was, the key to not being left behind was to have the conversation.

While in our cases the reaction from friends was 'we thought you wouldn't want to come', in some circles it's far more extreme. Many see the decision to not drink as a diss on the acceptability of their own actions. They feel defensive and don't like the fact that their norm has been challenged, so they set about getting things 'back to normal'. This can manifest as peer pressure or purposeful non-inclusion. Conform or leave. I mean, who needs friends like that?

Funnily enough, one of the things I realised early, and in fact found very easy, was to not judge other people's drunken behaviour. After all, I had been that person many, many times in the past. Who wants a judgemental eye over them when they're out enjoying themselves? My decision to not drink was all about me and my life and nothing to do with them and theirs. So go for it. Let your hair down. Blow off steam. Get locked. Do what you need to do and

I'll do what I need to do. As long as we're all happy with our choices, then there shouldn't be any issue.

At times, though, it was clear that some people weren't so happy with their choices. The conversation usually began well into the night, when someone would sidle up beside me and start asking questions. When you're not drinking, you get a lot of questions. People want to know why and they want to know how. Some are being polite, some are flabbergasted that it's actually possible, some are curious, some are nosy, some want the gory backstory and many more than I'd expected are genuinely interested. It turns out that they'd love to do it, but they just don't think they can.

Those conversations usually run like a script:

'So are you really off the booze?'

'Yep!'

'How come?'

'Well, I was going to take a break for a month but then I just kept going.'

'And how is it?'

'Surprisingly great, actually.'

'Amazing.'

'Yeah, I never thought I'd be a non-drinker.'

'Fair play. I'd love to try it, but I just know I wouldn't be able to.'

'Ah, you never know. I thought the same at the start. Might be worth a try sometime...'

Which brings us to another challenge: how to balance on the tightrope of telling people who ask about the amazing benefits and not becoming someone who tries to persuade others to join the alcohol-free club.

Almost everyone goes through an evangelical stage at the beginning. Just like any new obsession, we can't wait to share the benefits and bring everyone we know into the fold. At times I had to bite my cheeks and repeat in my head continuously, 'Shut up. Don't say it. They don't want to hear about it.' Most of the time I was successful, responding only when asked.

I would sometimes wonder about those people questioning me on nights out about how I did it. Were they waking up the next day thinking to themselves, 'FFS, Kate was on at me about giving up alcohol again. Would she ever back off?' Or maybe they were waking up with a sore head and thinking, 'FFS, I've done it again. I really need to take a break from alcohol like Kate.' Who knows?

I try hard not to push people into it (although this book may put paid to that), but knowing the benefits and the difference it has made to me and my life, I want everyone I love and care about to have the chance to experience an alcohol-free life – or how it feels to me, a free life. But I also know that sometimes the most persuasive argument is simply leading by example. When Kristian gave up drinking, he didn't extol the benefits and try to get everyone else onside. But we all saw the difference in him and through that our own journeys began. I see it with my sisters too. After years of jesting and taking the piss out of me for being so boring, they now occasionally give me little signals that maybe someday they would like to give it a go.

'I want to be like you when I grow up,' one birthday card message says.

'Can I borrow this?' holding up a quit lit book from my bookcase.

'The One Year No Beer daily email said that...'

Thoughts are breeding. Plans ruminating. Everyone takes their own trip in their own time when it comes to alcohol. In the four years since giving it up, I've had countless conversations about it, most instigated by other people. I've also written a couple of blog posts on it and a couple of articles. The first article, which appeared in the *Irish Independent*, sent a raft of new recruits to the One Year No Beer website, which confirmed my suspicions that there are plenty of people out there who want to break free from their own drinking habits. But the piece also received a couple of comments about how I was clearly an alcoholic before I gave up and why can't all the do-gooders back off and leave us alone to enjoy our pints in peace – which confirmed my suspicions that some people are extremely defensive about their relationship with alcohol and don't want anyone challenging the status quo. I get it. To be fair, I would have rolled my eyes at the article and quickly turned the page had I read it before I was ready to open my mind to the possibility of giving up. It's all about personal timing.

It's also all about learning what your triggers are.

On our return from Amsterdam at the very start of our first 30 days, I went through the kitchen cupboards. A third of a bottle of Bushmills single malt, an almost full bottle of Bombay Sapphire gin, an unopened bottle of very expensive Italian wine brought back from our summer holiday, a bottle of our standard weekend Rioja and a four-pack of Peroni.

I knew the whiskey wouldn't be a temptation, that the good wine would stay unopened and the gin was safe if I didn't have any tonic in the house, but the beers and Rioja had to go. I gave them away and kept the rest out of sight, waiting until the challenge was over. I knew that recognising triggers and habits was key to overcoming them. If I had a wobble on a Friday night, the beer or wine could easily be opened in a 'ah, fuck it' moment.

There was no symbolic pouring of drinks down the sink. Instead, I used the whiskey for cooking and the gin and prized bottle of wine remained, gathering dust. It was with a heavy heart that months later I handed the wine over to my sister, a lesson if ever there was one to stop saving special things for special occasions. Four years later, the gin is still there.

Fridays were a definite trigger for me. I associated the beginning of the weekend with a drink. It was a marker, the dividing line between the working week and time off. That first beer signified a clocking off, as obvious as punching out on a time clock on your way out the office door or factory floor. It was my transition from school and working week to weekend, a magic portal that shed the frantic always-on days and brought me to free time and a slower pace. That first sip was like a deep exhale.

The comedian Lee Mack tells a story in the introduction of *Try Dry*, another quit lit book. He and a friend went out for a drink shortly after he had decided to take a break from alcohol for a while. It had been a stressy day and he wanted something to release the pressure. His friend ordered a pint and he eyed it enviously, his lemonade looking sad and wanting beside it. As his pal lifted the glass to his lips and took a deep sip of the golden nectar, his whole body visibly relaxed. 'Ah, that's better,' he said, placing down his glass.

That's when the penny dropped for Mack. The release had absolutely nothing to do with the alcohol in his friend's glass, as it wouldn't have had any time to hit his system. His reaction had come from the symbolic going to the pub with a mate, ordering a drink and taking a sip of an ice-cold drink. His mind had clocked off, his body had relaxed. This man would therefore associate the pint of beer as his destressor, but actually it was all the other factors and nothing at all to do with the drink.

And so I realised that the key to my Friday nights was to have a different talisman and form a different habit. I began to buy in alcohol-free beers. There weren't many on the market at that time, but Erdinger had been around for years and was a pretty good substitute. Cold (alcohol-free) beer and posh crisps – a new Friday night association began.

But I didn't associate alcohol only with Friday nights – I associated it with stress relief. Who doesn't want a drink at the end of a particularly challenging day? I had used wine when the kids were young and the stress levels were through the roof. A friend with a big job in the city used gin and tonic. Every day of the working week, she would walk in her front door, exhausted from the commute and pressure of her job, and her husband would hand her a G&T at the bottom of the stairs, which she would then drink in the bath that he had run for her. That was her routine. She'd come back down the stairs 40 minutes later, tired but happy, having wiped the slate of her day clean. Could she cope with her stressful job without that drink at the end of each day? She didn't think so. Her belief was that her G&T marked the end of her work day and the beginning of a relaxing evening. My belief was that the hot bath, fresh pyjamas and dinner on the sofa would have done the trick just as well without the gin.

Now that I didn't have a drink as an option to relieve my stress, I needed to find something else. I turned to running. Exercise is the ultimate destressor. Instead of blocking out the stress like alcohol does, it allows your body and mind to deal with it. Midway into a run, the issue at hand wouldn't seem so bad after all and I'd start hatching plans on how to deal with it. Many a great idea and solution were thought of on the crest of a hill as the possibilities that minutes before had eluded me became endless and exciting. For me, running was key to the challenge of life's stresses. We can't escape the pressure, so we all need to find ways of dealing with it, and those ways can either be a positive or negative force on the rest of our lives.

The associations and triggers that most of us have with alcohol run deep. From Friday nights to stress relievers and celebrations to commiserations, every occasion and emotion is usually tied up with alcohol. How do you celebrate a birthday without a drink? Or toast a milestone without a glass of champagne? How do you relax at the weekend? Bond with friends? Escape from anxiety? Deal with grief? Or the one that took the longest for me to get my head around – how do you go out to a restaurant for a meal without ordering a bottle of wine?

For a long time, there seemed little point in bothering with the last one at all. I felt like the whole atmosphere would be ruined. And what was a steak without a hearty glass of red wine to bring out its flavour?

Over time, I learned that lots of people who give up drink actually find that their sense of smell and taste improve. Subtler flavours are picked up on and the meal becomes all about the food itself. It took me a while to come around to it, but it no longer bothers me at all that I'm now pairing a non-alcoholic beer with my ribeye.

One way that food became amplified for me, though, was through my sugar cravings. I've always had a sweet tooth, but suddenly my whole body was crying out for sugar, sugar and more sugar. In those first weeks my cravings for chocolate were worse than my cravings for wine. I'd read about others having the same experience, so it wasn't entirely unexpected. I decided to simply go with it. I would use sugar as my crutch to begin with, then wean myself off it once I had my other habits under control.

Replacing alcohol with sugar is commonplace and there's a scientific reason why. Our bodies convert alcohol to sugar, which causes a spike in our blood sugar levels. When we stop drinking our blood sugar levels can drop, which results in sugar cravings. Sometimes I would choose cake over a meal. I would always have chocolate stashed around the house in secret hiding places. (Parenting hack – always use the vegetable compartment of the fridge, no child ever goes there.) After a couple of months had passed and I knew that this was likely to be a longer-term experiment, I began to consciously cut back. I made energy balls with dates and cacao to give me a healthy sugar hit and blitzed up daily smoothies for the natural sweetness. It worked. Running, swimming and yoga led to cravings for nourishing foods. The healthier I became, the better I felt. The better I felt, the more I wanted to stay that way and

I felt less inclined to gorge on sweet treats. I was caught in a virtuous cycle instead of a vicious one. 'My body is a temple,' I would mutter to anyone rolling their eyes.

I've calmed down a bit since then. I eat more than my fair share of sugar and I order takeaways whenever I get the chance, but life is generally a healthy balance of real food and treat food. Everything in moderation, as they say (except alcohol, I would add!).

I was never fat exactly, but from secondary school to having kids, my weight had always fluctuated. In school I would put myself on calorie-counting diets and compare notes with friends on how many Ryvita crackers with cottage cheese we had eaten that day. I thought that I was fat when I was in college and into my early twenties, but photos tell a different story. I was definitely carrying a few too many extra pounds around for most of that time, but nothing extreme. I would frequently go on health kicks and fad diets. Juice fasts, the cabbage soup diet, 1,500 calories a day, no sugar, no carbs, no meat, all the meat – whatever was the next big thing, I was on it. And when I was on it, whatever I wasn't allowed to have became my obsession.

When I stopped eating carbs, the greatest loss to me was pasta. I loved it and would eat it every day if I could. Plus it was both cheap and easy. My absolute favourite was the spinach and ricotta tortellini made with fresh pasta that had recently hit supermarket shelves – the height of sophistication to twenty-something me in the 1990s. Now that I couldn't have them, I obsessed about them daily. I dreamed about them, fantasised about them, drooled over thoughts of them. Dripping with butter or fresh pesto sauce, a little black pepper and a glass of wine. I could not get the thoughts out of my head.

One Friday night, after what felt like months without touching them (but in fact was less than two weeks), I decided I would treat myself. Just the once and then back on the wagon. I went to the local supermarket and there they were on the shelf, waiting for me. But what's this? They were on special offer! Wrapped up in packs of two-for-one, I had no choice but to buy the deal, which I hotfooted it home with, thrilled but concerned. What would I do with the second packet?

I decided that I would limit my meal that night to half a packet. Which I did. And it tasted every bit as good as I had expected. But the portion was so small, I really should have cooked a little bit more ... I might as well do that now. I dropped a handful into fresh boiling water. But that only left a few in the packet, and sure what was the point in keeping them? So I threw in the rest and then ate a whole other bowl. I sat on the sofa, content and happy for a couple of hours.

But soon my mind turned to the other packet. Perhaps I should just get rid of it. By eating it. Then they would all be gone and I wouldn't have to think about them any more. I wrestled with eating/not eating the second packet until I got sick of listening to myself. I cooked up the whole lot and sat down to eat. I made it more than halfway through before I felt sick, disgusted at myself and full of self-loathing.

The irony, of course, was that I never would have eaten two packets of pasta if I hadn't been off carbs as part of my diet. The fact that I wasn't allowed pasta made pasta an obsession. Giving up anything can make you think that way, especially alcohol because it's such an ingrained part of our lives. It's sold to us as the fun-maker, risk-taker, life-liver, so giving that up is always going to be a challenge. For the first few weeks I thought about alcohol, talked about alcohol, even dreamed about alcohol constantly. During the tough times I would ask myself whether I was willing to give up the multitude of good stuff to go back to it. The answer was always a resounding no. The pros always far out-weighed the cons. As life went on and I began to get used to living without it, it became less and less of an obsession.

The key was replacing the 'treat' of alcohol with some-thing else. Sometimes it was sugar, sometimes it was exercise, sometimes it was sea swimming, sometimes it was a massage, sometimes it was alcohol-free beer. Filling the void that alcohol left in the early days meant that I didn't miss it so much.

Over the years, I have found that the challenges of giving up or taking a break from alcohol are different for everyone. Some find it easier than expected. Some are shocked to find that they can't do it. Some have lapses, then get straight back on the horse. Some don't even get to the starting line. The process depends on many factors – your relationship with alcohol in the first place, your friendship group, your personality, your situation, your history. But perhaps most of all, it depends on your supports.

Chapter 10

Supports

The truth is, I had no idea what I was getting into. I had innocently agreed to doing one month alcohol free, but I wasn't particularly happy about it. I liked drinking. I didn't have a problem with alcohol. Life was good. I had done a month off for Dry January before, so I knew I could do it. That wasn't the problem – the problem was that I had hated it. It was boring and depressing. When I wrote my 'Dear Dry January. I Hate You.' blog post, I meant every word. Let's go back to it in full, shall we?

> *Here's a tip for you. If anyone ever, ever asks you if you want to do Dry January with them – walk away. Don't look back, just keep on walking straight to that delicious bottle of cold beer calling out to you from its haven of loveliness.*
>
> *Because Dry January is a crock of shit. A farce that I have been stupidly suckered into.*
>
> *Of course, like me, you might be tempted after all those excesses at Christmastime. Might think it's just what your mind and body needs. Well, it isn't.*
>
> *Never have I been as bored, boring or depressed. Three weeks in and I am OVER it. Not only is it freezing cold and miserable – I am freezing cold and miserable. And sober.*
>
> *Call me an alcoholic, but life just isn't as much fun*

without alcohol. Friday night is the same as any other night. And Saturday is twice as depressing. Sipping on peppermint tea and watching a Downton Abbey *box set does not a weekend make.*

Naturally you will try to compensate for the lack of alcohol in your life with food. Chocolate ... ice cream ... cake ... chocolate ice cream cake... But it's not the same. And now you've lost the only thing you had keeping you going – the smugness of your 'my body is a temple' conversations.

Where's the fun? The sparkle? The release?

It's not that I can't do it. I'm just so BORED doing it.

Bored, bored, bored, bored, bored.

Bored.

Bored.

Expect a spectacular fall off the wagon come February. I've got some catching up to do.

Issues much there, Kate?

I cringe now reading that, but the comments that followed showed that I was far from alone in my feelings.

'This is me all over! I could have written this two years ago. I saw it through but hated every miserable wine-free evening. And Fridays were the absolute worst! I did begin to worry that I might be an alcoholic after my thoughts but having read this, I'm glad I'm not alone! Dry Jan can do one!'

'It's dull, eh? I gave up, the draw of gin was too strong.'

'I am so bored with it too. Saturday night drinking a cup of coffee is just not the same. Bring back alcohol, roll on Sunday!'

'I'm only drinking Friday and Saturday nights but to go cold turkey?! WHY would you want to do that! It'll just make you go crazy in February, and undo all the "good"!'

I wasn't lying. I did hate that month. But that's because I went into it completely wrong. I had no plan, and crucially, I had no supports in place. I didn't even know I needed them.

This time, it was different. Both Kristian and my brother Liam had shown me that taking a break was not only possible, but that it could be a good thing. Who knew? Instead of feeling deprived and miserable, they were happy and full of life. Seeing this meant that I went into the challenge with a positive mindset.

One of the greatest supports you can have when undertaking a challenge is other people taking the same path as you. Hearing from those who are one or two steps ahead of you can inspire you to get started or to keep going. I learned this first hand when my marriage broke up. I didn't want the expert advice or the sympathetic head tilts. I wanted people who had trod the muddy path already and got their boots dirty. People who had felt the heartache and the fear and had got through to the other side. I wanted their stories, their advice, their support. It's why I wrote my first book, *Untying the Knot*. I found it so hard to find those stories that I decided to tell my own for others coming after me.

Fortunately, when it comes to giving up alcohol the stories are plentiful and wildly positive. The One Year No Beer Facebook group gave me access to lots of stories from others who were on the same path as me – some further ahead, some with tragic backstories, some still fighting demons, but all with an overwhelming mood of positivity and inspiration. If I was feeling confused about the future or bored with the present, I could dip in for a quick shot of inspiration. It would inevitably leave me feeling stronger and more resolute. Even on days when I wasn't searching, a Facebook post would pop up in my feed and remind me that thousands of other people around the globe were leading better, more fulfilling lives because they'd ditched the booze. Every post topped up my belief that life could be better without alcohol.

But that wasn't all I had. Not only did I have an online support group on tap whenever I needed a little pep talk, I also had a real one. Going to family events where up to four out of eight of us weren't drinking was a gift in itself. It normalised the process and took the pressure off.

Of course, the person who made the biggest difference was Aodhan. And likewise for him having me. The fact that we each had a partner to lean on in social situations and that we could talk through the whole process with each other had a massive impact on the experience for both of us.

'Isn't it mad that...' one of us would begin as we unpicked another long-held belief about alcohol.

Isn't it mad that we don't feel comfortable with friends without a drink?

Isn't it mad that we actually poison our bodies until we are physically sick?

Isn't it mad that we spend 60 years of our lives drinking?

Isn't it mad that people get so defensive about alcohol?

Isn't it mad that people don't know that drinking causes cancer?

Isn't it mad the amount of money we all spend on alcohol?

Isn't it mad that alcohol is the only drug that people don't congratulate you for giving up?

Isn't it mad that giving up drink is considered such an extraordinary thing to do?

Well it is, isn't it? We found it fascinating and could talk about it for hours together. The ultimate reformed drinkers. Thankfully, no one else had to listen to us because we had each other. But the psychology of why we drink is a deep and intriguing study. There's personality, family, history, culture and environmental factors all at play.

We became students in a class of two with the internet as our professor. It didn't take long for us to stumble on other resources that delved into the same subject. There were sobriety schools and sobriety toolkits, there were government guides and free ebooks, there were chat rooms and Facebook groups. And there were thousands and thousands of corny memes.

I would dip in and out, finding favourites and nodding sagely at the advice or experience that mirrored mine. But a lot of them focused on addiction and recovery and I knew that wasn't me. I wasn't a problem drinker, I was a 'normal' drinker. I could have a glass of wine without drinking the bottle. I could have beers in the fridge without touching them for a week. I didn't get difficult or argumentative or messy when I was drunk. I never drank in the morning or was tempted by the hair of the dog. I never got drunk alone. Drink didn't cause me direct issues with work, relationships, money or health (other than hangovers). I was the same sort of drinker as the majority of my friends, family and acquaintances. But I was still a drinker. And there was no escaping the fact that I, along with all those friends, family and acquaintances, was drink dependent because I needed it to socialise and I couldn't imagine life without it.

Hello Sunday Morning, Hip Sobriety and The Tempest all spoke to me with blog posts on The Fear of Socialising without Booze, Why You Shouldn't Rely on Alcohol

When You Are Stressed, What Happens When You Stop Drinking Alcohol and 9 Reasons the Term 'Alcoholic' Should Die Already.

Holly Whitaker from Hip Sobriety is a leading light in the world of sobriety. She's honest, raw and funny with great advice to bestow on all of us. Her journey began in 2012 when she was living what from the outside looked like a charmed life: a director at a hot San Francisco start-up, lots of hip friends and a full social calendar. But in actual fact, her life was chaotic, she was unhappy and was drinking to extreme levels ('a few bottles of wine or a few pints of Jameson most nights').

When I first read her background, I almost clicked away. It was way out of my league and she had a level of drinking that I would have categorised as alcoholic, not one that I could relate to myself. But she also wrote that if she could give up drink then anyone could, and that struck me. She believed that the sooner you start, the easier it is and that you don't have to hit rock bottom to change your relationship with alcohol. What I liked best was her simple but clear-cut response to something so sprawling and emotive. Especially this:

> Am I an alcoholic? is the wrong question. You don't
> need an online questionnaire to determine whether or
> not you have a drinking problem. The only questions
> you need to ask are (1) whether drinking alcohol is

getting in the way of your dreams in this one life you
have been given, and (2) how much longer you're
willing to settle for that.

I presume that if you're reading this book, the answers to 1 and 2 are something along the lines of 'I think so' and 'I'm not sure'. And that's okay. It takes time for these ideas to ruminate and take root.

Hello Sunday Morning is an Australian not-for-profit organisation dedicated to helping people who want to change their relationship with alcohol. Their social media accounts are filled with positivity and people embracing their sober weekends. But as always, it's the personal stories that pack the most punch. If you ever need inspiration to keep going or confirmation that you're on the right path, reading a few quick posts about other people's personal experience usually does the trick. There were women talking about how their mood swings stopped, their minds became sharper, their physical and mental health improved. There were men who wrote about becoming better husbands and fathers and finding themselves fitter and stronger than they had been in years. And there were lots of Whys.

'I wanted to be the woman who could enjoy the natural pleasures of summer – long hot nights, ocean swims, warm early mornings – without diluting them with alcohol,' wrote Vari. I thought about that a lot. Why is it that when we are on holiday, already relaxed and happy, we feel the need to take a drink? I thought back to the many holidays I'd spent lying on sun loungers by the pool and thinking a cold beer was called for. Was it? The idea of it was appealing. Those first few sips were amazing. But the after-effect, if I was completely honest with myself, was a bit of a dulled tiredness. A sparkling ice-cold soda would have done a better job if I hadn't been indoctrinated by the power of our drinking culture.

There were also plenty of personal challenges on the sites, from dealing with grief and stress without alcohol as a crutch to friendships and marriages. A woman named Samantha wrote:

> I have NEVER moved through a life crisis without numbing the pain. I have NEVER properly dealt with these tough painful human emotions. I have NEVER processed properly shock, grief and anger. To do so has been a wonderful experience – and I think part of the reason why I have gone through the experience. They say everything does happen for a reason – and a big one for me was to learn how to do this thing called 'life' without turning to drinking and escaping the hard stuff.

That made me look at my own life crises in a different light. Numbing myself on the day my father died, drinking too much as my marriage fell apart, losing my job and looking for solace in a glass (or five) of red wine.

The stories were real and varied and covered every topic that I had struggled with or revelled in. It was deeply supportive to know that others had taken this path too, and although less travelled, it was all the more wonderous for that reason.

Along with the websites came the books. Who knew that quit lit was a thing? There were books about addiction and recovery written by former alcoholics who'd reached lows that were almost impossible to climb out of, but there were also books written by 'normal' drinkers who had let things get a little out of hand. There were books about the psychology of alcohol and books with step-by-step instructions on giving up for 30 days.

I read *The Unexpected Joy of Being Sober* by Catherine Gray after I'd already been alcohol free for about a year. It affirmed my whole experience of giving up. It was all about the positives, from energy and productivity to happiness and health. She writes:

> *I found myself with dozens more hours in the week, heaps more energy, £23,000 more money over four years, deepened friendships, revived family relationships, better skin, a tighter body, tanned legs for the first time ever, the ability to sleep for eight uninterrupted hours, a bone-deep sense of well-being, a totally turned-around positive outlook and an infinitely more successful career. What's not to like?!*

Indeed.

Author Clare Pooley 'never expected to find herself an overweight, depressed, middle-aged mother of three who was drinking more than a bottle of wine a day, and spending her evenings Googling "Am I an alcoholic?"'. She writes in *The Sober Diaries*, 'I learned that if you drink to blur all the difficult things in life, you blur all the good stuff too.' Her story is witty and relatable and provided an easy reminder that I was on the right path.

Annie Grace is widely regarded as the queen of quit lit. Her book *This Naked Mind* came out in 2015. In it, she not only gives her own story but weaves in psychological, neurological, cultural, social and industry factors to provide insight into the reasons why we drink. Her hard-hitting quotes are plentiful.

One point that Grace says is raised in many non-drinking discussions is this: 'Our society not only encourages drinking – it takes issue with people who don't drink.' Alcohol is the only drug that you have to apologise for when giving it up. Our society is deeply distrustful of people who choose not to drink. In the early days I spent a lot of time apologising for or embarrassed about my choice. It took at least a year before I could say 'I don't drink' without shame, let alone any hint of pride.

I remember the first time I said 'I don't drink' out loud. We were at a restaurant and someone was about to pour me a glass of wine.

'Oh, I'm fine, thanks. I don't drink.'

It just popped out of my mouth, unexpected and shocking. For me at least. I hadn't thought about saying it before the words just tumbled out. I'd never heard myself say it out loud before. It sounded strange, yet natural.

'Do you not?' she asked. I missed the rest of her reaction because I was repeating those same words over and over in my head, rolling them around like a precious stone I was examining.

'I don't drink. I don't drink. I *don't* drink. I don't *drink*. *I* don't drink.'

It had taken over a year to get to that point. In part possibly because I wasn't ready to believe that I wouldn't drink again and partly because I wasn't ready for other people's reactions. In my head I wasn't a non-drinker or a teetotaller – those labels came with too much baggage. I was simply not drinking *at the moment*.

Up to that point, 'I don't drink' had always equated to 'I am dull'. I might as well have worn a warning sign around my neck telling people to steer clear of the weirdo in the corner. But some time over those past 12 months, unbeknownst to myself, I had shed the shame and was ready to own it. My subconscious had made the switch before I had consciously made the decision. But there I was, a non-drinker.

I don't drink.

I tried the label on for size and found that in fact I quite liked it. Instead of it sounding dull, it seemed almost exotic. In a world where everyone around you is drinking, to not drink is an act of rebellion, like not having a Facebook account or refusing to own a mobile phone.

Annie Grace's book is a big read, but fascinating for opening doors of perception that you'd never realised were even there. It helped to lift the veil for me, revealing that there was so much cultural belief ingrained in me that it would take both strength of character and new knowledge to remain a non-drinker in a drinking world.

✳ ✳ ✳

Things have come a long way in the four years since I've given up drink. In pubs, my whispered 'Do you have any alcohol-free beers?' would be met with a quizzical frown or 'Um, we might have an Erdinger somewhere – let me just check.' The barman would then disappear into the back or onto his hands and knees to pull the last remaining bottle of warm non-alcoholic beer from the recesses of the bar's dusty foundations. He would then proudly hold the bottle aloft like Harrison Ford in *Indiana Jones and the Last Crusade* showing off his Holy Grail. 'Found it!' he would declare delightedly. I would then slink back to my seat, hoping no one had been watching the display.

Nowadays I can walk into a bar or restaurant anywhere in the country and confidently order one, sometimes from a selection.

'We have Paulaner or Heineken o.o.'

'We have Erdinger or Open Gate Pure Brew.'

'We have an IPA, Peroni or Cobra.'

Last year Aodhan and I went for a pre-gig dinner in a casual Dublin restaurant. When we asked the question, the young waiter serving us gave us a list of three to choose from and then described each of them, which one he preferred and why. It was one of the first times alcohol-free drinks had been at the centre of a discussion on taste with any staff I'd come into contact with in bars, shops or restaurants. And it was nice. Really nice. Here was someone who understood that taste matters even when your beer has no alcohol in it. He valued our choice and totally got it. And he was only in his early twenties. A hint of things to come, perhaps.

Almost every big brewery is now producing alcohol-free beers and it makes a world of difference. I'm not sure I'll ever break free from that association of having a cold beer to switch off, but it turns out I don't have to.

Open Gate Pure Brew is now my tipple of choice. I'll have that first sip that flicks the switch just like Lee Mack's friend's pint of the real stuff did. It doesn't matter whether the alcohol is in there or not. I enjoy both the taste and the experience. Having a bottle of alcohol-free beer feels exactly the same as having a bottle of normal beer. But after a couple, I've had enough – there's no need to keep drinking them. Plus I don't suffer any ill effects.

We dabbled with alcohol-free wines too but have never

found one worth drinking. It can be nice to have a bottle on the table for a special meal, but they are always disappointing, which only leaves you wondering about the real thing. So we stopped bothering.

Sparkling wines, however, are a different story. Coming up to our second Christmas, we discovered that our local supermarket was selling a couple of different versions that were surprisingly good, including a prosecco that wasn't too sweet and perfect for toasting or celebrating when served chilled in a champagne glass. You can now find 'no-secco' in Tesco and plenty of other options in most supermarkets and off licences.

It seems we weren't the only ones to discover them. The following Christmas they were sold out in all the local shops and the managers were having trouble sourcing stock. As new alcohol-free options come to market, I get genuinely excited. For one thing it gives me another drink to try, but it also tells me that we aren't alone. There are lots of others on the same bandwagon.

'Look at this!' I squealed with embarrassing levels of excitement back at the start as I showed Aodhan the paper. The *Sunday Times* 'What's Hot' list included a new drink called Seedlip. Minimally packaged in a thick glass bottle with an artistic label, it was a thing of beauty. It claimed to be 'the world's first non-alcohol distilled spirit'. It was described as alcohol-free gin and the price tag was, well, reassuringly expensive.

That Christmas we went to my brother Liam's house for drinks. The fire was glowing, the fairy light twinkling and the gin and tonics flowing. 'Would you like one of these?' he asked, holding aloft the perfect bottle.

I couldn't have been more excited by a drink and don't think I ever have been. (Other than that first bottle of Moët I ever tasted. Or that bottle of expensive Sancerre I had in that posh London restaurant. Or the Brunello I bought as a gift to myself in Italy. Or the time when I was 16 and someone gave me a sip of their Malibu and pineapple...) Anyway, it was a thrill. It was grown-up and complex and made me feel like part of the gang. With Fever Tree tonic and a slice of lime, I couldn't have been more content. It tasted every bit as good as a 'real' gin and tonic and it made me feel included.

In the past 12 months the alcohol-free drinks trend has really taken off, with Tesco now hosting an entire Zero Zone. There are beers, ciders, sparkling wines, gins and more. And it's only getting bigger. As I write this, the alcohol-free version of Guinness is now getting ready to hit our shelves (albeit with a bit of a bumpy ride), having been in development for over four years.

Cheers!

* * *

Exercise was the first step towards filling my life with alternative activities that didn't involve alcohol. As I began to plan and do new things, my life started to open up and became more full and more rewarding than it had been in years. I ran, I swam, I did yoga, I went to art galleries and plays, I played with my kids instead of brushing them off because I was tired, I went hiking and exploring, I wrote, I read, I baked, I spent money on massages and facials that would previously have been spent in the pub. I lived life to the full and instead of feeling like I was missing out, I felt like I had won the life lottery. I had been given a second chance. I had been gifted the opportunity to live a more rewarding, more present, more fulfilling existence. It wasn't so much smugness as gratitude. I just felt incredibly lucky.

The late, great A.A. Gill was a reformed alcoholic who gave up drink aged 30. His quotes and writing about his journey to sobriety are bountiful, but the one that always stuck with me was one I read long before I even considered giving up myself. 'I don't feel I've been cheated of anything … I gave up [alcohol] when I was still young, so it was like being offered the next life. It was the real Willy Wonka golden ticket, I got a really good deal.'

When I first read that, it made sense to me for an alcoholic like him to feel that way about drink. But now I know the same is true for any drinker. He also said, 'What started out as the key, ended as the jail.' Again, I think many of us can relate to that even though we may not be considered alcoholics.

(Completely unrelated: Gill, who was a restaurant critic, also wrote one of my favourite-ever lines about food: 'Pasta is eaten by happy smiley people having fun with people they love or fancy and are about to shag. Noodles are eaten by people who have no friends.' I've always loved pasta.)

Andy Ramage of the One Year No Beer movement agrees that it's all about the change in mindset – that taking a break from alcohol is not about giving up something, but rather more about giving you the chance to gain a clear advantage in life. 'The conventional wisdom that yells "we need alcohol to have fun, be a success and live a full life" is wrong,' he states. Anyone who has taken an extended break from alcohol is likely to agree.

✶ ✶ ✶

They say it takes 21 days to break a habit, but that's not strictly true. It depends on the person – and the habit. What *is* certain, though, is that the longer you do something, the easier it becomes. So the longer you stick with giving up alcohol, the less you have to think about it. But breaking a habit is also about forming new habits. The two really go hand in hand. Instead of watching TV and eating biscuits every Monday night, you go for a walk with Joan. Instead of smoking a cigarette after lunch, you chew a piece of gum. Instead of taking a drink when you're stressed, you have a bath. Before long you associate

Monday nights with walking with Joan, lunchtimes with gum and relaxing with baths. It sounds simplistic, but that's the essence of what happens.

The problem is that drinking is so ingrained in so many parts of our lives and emotions that it's not like breaking down or building up just one habit – it's like breaking down your whole life. What I found, though, is that practice really does make perfect, so every pub trip I made it through, every party or gathering I attended without drinking all bolstered my belief that I could do it. It also interrupted the habit of ordering a drink just because I was out. It made me stop and think. Likewise on a Friday night at home or after a stressful day, the more I actively broke the habit of automatically reaching for a drink without even thinking about it, the easier it became to form new habits. Becoming aware of those triggers and having substitutions in place made the switch much easier.

All these things listed here were in my survival tool-kit, whether I realised it at the time or not. They are the reasons why I not only found those first 30 days relatively easy, but that I chose to continue to 90 days, 100 days, 365 days and onwards.

Chapter 11

State of the Nation

In theory it seemed like a great idea.

I had received a call earlier in the year asking if I would be interested in speaking at a corporate event to share my story of giving up alcohol. Of course I would! It would be directly after New Year, just in time for Dry January. Fantastic! There would be talks on mental health, pensions and safety at work. Sounds brilliant! And it will be for a couple of hundred construction workers. Oh.

Tough crowd, I thought to myself, but sure, why not? I mean, it's very small-minded of me to think that construction workers would be any less open to going sober than other types of employees. I'd just put on my big girl pants, practise the hell out of it and see who it connected with on the day. I wasn't selling anything, I wasn't lecturing them, I was just telling my own story. How bad could it be? (We all know where this is going...)

On the morning of the talk, I drove deep into the Irish heartlands. In the small country town Google Maps had brought me to, there was a community hall and outside in their work boots and jackets stood a group of men on their smoke break. I knew in that moment that this was going to be a harder sell than I'd anticipated. But still, I was game.

'Come on, Kate, you can do this. It's not going to be for everybody but there's bound to be a few in the audience who are at that post-Christmas-sick-of-booze point. It'll all be over soon...'

I walked through the intimidating crowd at the door in my high-heeled boots and fake confidence and got my laptop ready. But time was running over on the event, so as the last speaker before me finished everyone stood up to head out to lunch. There was shuffling and confusion as they were told that there was actually one more speaker before lunch, so they were all brought reluctantly back inside to their seats again.

To listen to me. Telling them they shouldn't be drinking.

It was the worst start imaginable, but I powered on. As the wall of silence grew, I realised that I was out of my depth. I was not the right speaker for this crowd and this crowd was not the right audience for me.

My mouth dried up and I reached a shaky hand out to take a drink. The plastic cup shook so much I couldn't get it to my mouth, so I had to put it down and carried on, not only parched with thirst but knowing that now they all knew how nervous I was. The facade was broken. I wrapped it up as fast as I possibly could and collected my belongings. On the way out, one of the guys kindly told me that I had done really well and that the talk had been very interesting. We both knew it wasn't true, but I appreciated the sentiment all the same.

And then, horror of horrors, I had to do it all over again a second time for the next group. Once again, I was hit with timing from hell – I was the last slot on the Friday afternoon of a two-day event. Two men at the front of this audience decided that they had had enough. They began to snigger into their hands and make private jokes to each other about getting out and going for a pint. I tried to direct my next point at them, smiling as nonchalantly as I could, but they stared me back out of it and continued to chat between themselves. There was no coming back from it.

I raced through the remainder of the presentation in half the time allotted to me and ran out to my waiting car. If anything was ever going to drive me to drink again, it was that talk about giving up drink.

It took me a long time to recover from it. My confidence was shot and I couldn't escape the feelings of shame and failure every time I thought back on it. I have appeared on TV and been interviewed for podcasts and radio many times. It's always been a little nerve wracking, but ultimately enjoyable. Why was this time so different? I berated myself for not being better and for trying to do it at all. But in the end, I just had to accept that these were not my people. It wasn't their fault and it wasn't mine. I could have given that same talk to a group of women in their thirties and forties and had a completely different reaction. And likewise, a thirty-something guy could have delivered the same message at the event and been an inspiration.

But the real lesson for me was that not everyone wants to hear the message about alcohol. Not everyone is ready to deal with their relationship with it. And even when they are, it takes the right message at the right time by the right person in the right way to really make an impact.

* * *

Why do we drink? Good question. There is, of course, not just one answer. There is a variety of factors at play when it comes to us picking up a drink – psychological, social, environmental. We drink to escape, we drink to get drunk, we drink to be sociable, we drink because that's what people do to celebrate or commiserate or bond, we drink to enjoy ourselves, we drink to soothe ourselves, we drink because everyone else is drinking, we drink because that's what we've learned to do.

A study by Mulford and Miller published in 1960 divided each of the factors at play into either 'personal-effect motives' or 'social-effect motives'. Personal motives, or 'drinking to cope', would include drinking to escape negative emotions such as stress or trauma (negative rein-forcement). Social motives would be drinking to be more sociable, to fit in, to celebrate (positive reinforcement).

Personally, I think you could go further. If we drink among friends to enjoy ourselves and feel more comfort-able socialising (positive reinforcement), aren't we simply escaping our feelings of discomfort about being sober in that social setting (negative reinforcement)? In which case, even the positive comes from the negative.

Essentially, every factor comes down to being true to who you really are in any given situation and how you cope with difficult feelings. This line from the author Glennon Doyle from her book *Love Warrior* wraps it up nicely: 'Ah, yes. An Afgo.' 'Excuse me?' 'Another fucking growth opportunity.'

When I discovered you could relax and feel like you fit in with nothing more than an alcohol-free beer, I wondered why we all don't just drink them. But of course there's one thing missing, isn't there? The 'buzz' you get from alcohol.

But what is the buzz and how long does it last? For most people, it goes something like this:

Stage one: You begin to feel more relaxed. (First drink.)

Stage two: It's likely that you'll be more talkative, euphoric and less inhibited. (Second or third drink.) This is why most of us drink, to get to this magic point. But that point rarely lasts because drinking alcohol makes you want to drink more alcohol. So you swiftly move on to…

Stage three: You may start slurring your speech. You probably still feel happy. You don't realise that you're drunk. You may begin to stumble. You may feel sick. Your reactions are slower.

Stage four: If you get to this stage, you may experience blackouts and confusion. Your judgement is severely impaired. You may vomit.

Stage five: You become unresponsive to your surroundings. You may lose consciousness. Your situation may be life threatening.

So maybe having just one drink or two every so often is the answer? Maybe, but that's definitely easier said than done for most of us. Personally, I find it's easier to live by the 100 Per Cent Rule. When I learned to push through the difficult feelings of my own 'Afgo', I began to feel more confident in myself and who I truly am. Plus now I'd much rather choose real happy over alcohol-induced happy when I'm out. My magic moment now lasts for the whole evening. Plus sober belly laughs are the best.

But perhaps not everyone drinks to excess. Perhaps the majority of drinkers stop after one or two. At times I wondered whether Aodhan and I were operating in a bubble. I drank, my friends drank, my family drank, Aodhan drank, his friends drank, his family drank. The level of alcohol consumption between us all was similar, but was that simply because we moved in similar circles, like gravitating to like? Were we the norm or the outliers? Were most other people sipping on a glass of wine with their meals and taking or leaving it the rest of the time? Would they be appalled by the habits of our friendship groups?

I had occasionally been to swanky drinks parties where the host would carry a single glass of champagne around with her for the night, checking in on her guests and, gasp, seemingly enjoying herself. Was this normal? Was this how other people operated?

The facts, unfortunately, tell me otherwise.

Binge drinking is defined by health experts, including the World Health Organization (WHO), as having six or more standard drinks at the one sitting – the equivalent of just three pints. Surprised? You betcha.

The 2015 Healthy Ireland Survey reported that four out of 10 drinkers in Ireland binge drink to harmful levels on a monthly basis, with over one-fifth doing so on a weekly basis. Surprised? Not at all.

The WHO's 2016 Global Status Report on Alcohol and Health backed up these figures, reporting that almost half of all drinkers in Ireland had engaged in binge drinking in the previous month. This puts Ireland in the top six of the 194 countries studied. Not a league table you want to be at the top of, really.

It seems that we are a nation of binge drinkers. Unable to sip on a single drink for an evening like some of our Mediterranean counterparts, we drink it all in one go in case it runs out. The 2014 National Alcohol Diary Survey reports that a massive 75% of all alcohol consumed in Ireland in 2013 was done so as part of a binge drinking session.

So it seems that Aodhan and I had been 'normal' drinkers. We drank to excess in the same way as almost half the drinking population in the country. That's a hell of a lot of people getting pissed up at the weekend.

'So what?' you might ask. So everything.

Unfortunately, drinking isn't a harmless pastime. Whether we like it or not, alcohol is a drug that negatively impacts every area of society. As drinkers, we don't want to hear this.

'Sure, it's only a couple of drinks.'

'Yes, but *I* don't have a problem.'

'I'm only harming myself, not anyone else, so leave me alone.'

'It won't happen to me.'

'Oh for God's sake, lighten up.'

I understand the thought process. This was my reaction in the past whenever I heard, saw or read anything about the impact of alcohol. I didn't want to know. I didn't want to think about it.

But here are some of the undisputed facts around alcohol. They probably thought it wouldn't happen to them either.

Thirty-eight per cent of all road deaths in Ireland are related to alcohol.

When I was in my early twenties, a local guy was knocked down in a hit and run on a quiet back road of my town. He was coming home from a night out. The driver probably was too – maybe that's why he or she didn't stop. The twenty-something, fit, athletic young man was cut down in his prime, paralysed from the waist down. The driver was never caught, but they will be living with that knowledge forever. Two lives ruined.

Even if you would never, ever drink drive, one in two pedestrians killed on Irish roads had consumed alcohol.

And who hasn't walked home from a night out at some stage in their lives?

Research by the Road Safety Authority published in 2019 also found that 75% of fatalities between the hours of 10 p.m. and 6 a.m. (off-peak) had a positive toxicology for alcohol.

Shockingly, suicide is the leading cause of death among young Irish men aged 15 to 24. And alcohol is a factor in half of them.

According to Alcohol Action Ireland:

> *Alcohol can reduce inhibitions enough for an individual to act on suicidal thoughts which they might never have done if not under the influence of alcohol. The World Health Organization (WHO) has estimated that the risk of suicide when a person is currently abusing alcohol is eight times greater than if they were not abusing alcohol.*

Dr Bobby Smyth is a consultant child and adolescent psychiatrist and a board member of Alcohol Action Ireland. In a 2013 *Irish Times* article, he wrote some of the most crucial and telling information that I have read on the subject:

> *The majority of young men who take their own lives are intoxicated at the time. While we may choose to believe that people take alcohol in order to complete the act of suicide this is rarely the case.*

Many of these young men and women have no history of suicidal behaviour. While we cannot know what exactly is going on in the mind of someone who completes suicide, we can at least learn from those who survive serious attempts. As a psychiatrist I have met many such people.

Next, he lays out what often leads up to such a tragic event:

The typical sequence of events goes as follows. You are in bad form for whatever reason, often to do with relationships. You decide to have a few drinks to help you forget about it, as our culture encourages you to do. It doesn't work.

You think about it even more. You do or say something, perhaps in an effort to sort out the relationship problem; but you are drunk, so it doesn't work out so well. You feel worse. You decide to drink some more.

As you get more drunk, the future is foreshortened. You are impulsive and have greater difficulty thinking of solutions. Life seems suddenly impossible and unbearable. Suicide begins to look like a solution and in your disinhibited, disorientated state you act on it.

As a mother of teens, I read this and my blood ran cold.

Interestingly, one of the comments underneath this piece reads:

> *I for one can't stand the preachiness of articles above. Dislike the mothering attitude the state has taken with regard to alcohol. Ultimately drink is not an issue unless you let it be, a bit of cop on is all that's needed.*

If ever you doubted the hold that alcohol has over our society, that's it right there.

I might as well machine gun you down with some of the other facts while we're here.

Twenty-five per cent of deaths of young men aged 15 to 39 in Ireland are due to alcohol.

Alcohol is a common feature in crimes such as public order offences, assault and murder as well as rape and sexual assault, and there has been a large increase in all alcohol-related crime since the early 1990s.

Women are more vulnerable to tissue damage, cirrhosis of the liver and alcohol dependence. Alcoholic liver disease (ALD) rates are increasing rapidly in Ireland and the greatest level of increase is among 15- to 34-year-olds, who historically had the lowest rates of liver disease.

Among Irish women, four in 10 (40.9%) alcohol-related cancer deaths were due to breast cancer between 2001 and 2010.

Almost two-thirds (63.9%) of males and half (51.4%) of females started drinking alcohol before the age of 18 years.

Harmful drinking is highest among the 18- to 24-year-old age group (at 75%).

One in 11 children's lives are being negatively impacted by alcohol.

Every day, 1,500 beds in overcrowded hospitals are occupied by people with alcohol-related problems, costing the taxpayer €1.5 billion for alcohol-related discharges from hospital.

In fact, if you add together the cost of all the alcohol-related spend by the state on health, social care, crime and the justice system, the figure is closer to €4 billion.

These are big figures and it can be hard to get your head around them, but essentially this is money and resources and personnel that could be deployed elsewhere. So what it actually translates to is your granddad lying on a hospital trolley for 48 hours or your mum waiting a year for an operation or the ambulance not reaching your baby in time. Imagine what could be done with those billions if we didn't all drink to the levels that we do in our culture.

When you look at the money involved in all aspects of the alcohol industry, it is mind boggling. According to the Statista website's worldwide information on alcoholic drinks, direct global revenue in 2020 from the alcohol industry was worth €1.2 trillion. The US is the top revenue driver at €196 billion, the UK fifth at €53 billion and Irish figures are estimated at €5 billion.

'Not bad!' you might think when you look at us compared to the other two. Until you get into the per capita numbers: €1,008.43 per person for Ireland, €781.04 for the UK and €594.24 for the US. The only good news is that it's coming down at a faster rate year on year than the others.

Drinks industry reports say that 'together, manufacturers, distillers, brewers, pubs, off-licences, restaurants, hotels the length and breadth of the country generate €2.3 billion in revenue for the Exchequer every year'. On the face of it, it's obviously not in the government's interest to reduce these figures and the lobbyists within the industry have a powerful voice, so the revenue keeps growing, regardless of the wider cost to our society.

But if we are indeed seeing €2.3 billion in revenue from alcohol-related industries, it's still a lot less than the €4 billion in estimated costs to the state from alcohol-related issues.

*　*　*

If the power behind the alcohol industry was ever in doubt, the phased release from Covid-19 lockdown in the summer of 2020 made it very clear. Here we were, in the middle of a global pandemic, and we were actively giving the green light for people to enter a busy room to consume a substance that breaks down decision-making capabilities and removes social inhibitions. Why? Meanwhile, many businesses remained closed, childcare services were only just resuming and maternity services were left in limbo.

Journalist Jennifer O'Connell wrote an article in the *Irish Times* asking, 'Pubs are a Covid-19 risk. Why are we rushing to reopen them?' Indeed. It made no sense.

In those early months of lockdown there were rules around when and where and for how long you could drink, and pubs that did not serve meals could not open. Many people were angry about this, not least the Licensed Vintners Association. Some people wanted drink available in the usual formats, whenever and wherever they wanted. Others were of the 'safety first' opinion – let's just wait and see. The publicans understandably wanted their livelihoods back. The government wanted to please everyone. The resulting rules that were made around the issue seemed strange and nonsensical.

I'm no expert, but I'd imagine alcohol lobbyists are far more powerful than, say, childcare or maternity rights lobbyists, if such things even exist. To me it seemed that too much time and effort were being placed on something that was on the discussion table for all the wrong reasons. How many hours of consultations and planning were taken up with this one topic?

The decision to reopen the pubs during 2020 was not just about letting us go out and have a drink, or even about people's jobs and livelihoods. It is far more wide reaching and complex than that. It's to do with money, and industry, and, yes, public opinion. As a society we are simply so far under the spell of alcohol that we don't see it for what it is. A survey in TheJournal.ie in September 2020, as the second wave was taking hold, asked, 'Do you think "wet" pubs should be allowed to reopen this month?' Forty-eight per cent of respondents chose 'yes, absolutely'.

By mid-September 2020, a lot of pubs and restaurants were open but many pregnant women still could not have their partner attend antenatal appointments with them. This felt to me like supports for other areas of society during the early days of the crisis were damaged because of our obsession with alcohol.

However, when it comes to drinking and Ireland, there are both positive and negative forces to focus on. While the bad news is that illnesses such as liver disease are significantly on the rise and the amount of alcohol that we are drinking is one of the highest in the world (2015 figures from the Health Research Board show that people who drink in Ireland are consuming the equivalent of 46 bottles of gin or vodka, 130 bottles of wine or 498 pints of beer each in a year), there is hope for the next generations.

One Saturday afternoon during the summer of 2019, I was walking through my hometown. The sun was out, the shades were on and there was that promise of freedom in the air. As I passed the local off-license, two young men came out carrying a box of beer. Early twenties, shorts and T-shirts, I assumed they were off to a barbecue. So far, so normal. But then I noticed that the box they were carrying was full of non-alcoholic beer. I did a double take and forced myself not to pull out a microphone and start interviewing them there and then. 'Keep walking. Leave them alone. Don't be the crazy lady,' I muttered to myself, taking quick sidelong glances as I passed.

Young people's attitude to drink is changing. It's slow and it's in pockets, but it is happening. Maybe it's the wellness trend, maybe it's social media, maybe it's awareness and education, but there's a definite move towards choosing not to drink, and that choice is becoming more normalised.

Earlier that year I had been asked to go on to the Ray D'Arcy Show on RTÉ to be part of a panel discussing going sober. There was the *Irish Times* Health Correspondent Paul Cullen, representing the expert view; me, representing women and middle-aged folk; and a young man named Bobby Moran who had decided to take a break from alcohol in his early twenties. When we came onto the stage in front of the live studio audience, there was a frisson of excitement in the air. The ads were airing and as we sat down the audience didn't know what the piece would be about. There were smiles and chatter all around the room.

And then we were live. The host introduced the segment and welcomed us all and the room instantly changed. A silent wall went up between us and them. Arms were folded and an uncomfortable silence emanated from the crowd. Paul talked about the dangers of alcohol that we are all so blinded to. I spoke about my own experience. But it was Bobby who saved us. This unassuming young twenty-something guy spoke of drinking his way through college like everyone else around him. He recognised that life, his great love of sport and his goals were slipping away from him and he wanted to get a handle on things before it was too late. He knew that he couldn't do it while he was still drinking, so he stopped. He wasn't sure whether it would be a year, two, five or forever, but life was good because of it. I chatted to his girlfriend in the green room afterwards and she was delighted with the change in him. Everyone loved Bobby. It was hard not to.

The most recent Health Behaviour in School-aged Children study (the HBSC), which collects data every four years on our children's wellbeing, social environments and health behaviours, contains lots of worrying data. Between 2014 and 2018, it showed a 9% increase for 15- to 17-year-old girls within the high- and middle-social class groups when asked if they had drank in the last 30 days.

But it also shows an overall decrease from 20% to 17% of 12- to 17-year-olds who had an alcoholic drink in the past 30 days.

A decrease of 10% to 6% of those who were drunk in the past 30 days.

A decrease from 21% to 17% of those reporting to have ever been 'really drunk'.

And a modest increase of 6% in the number of school-aged children who have never drunk alcohol across all social classes.

So perhaps change is slowly creeping in for our children. Maybe by the time our children's children are in school it will be socially acceptable for them not to drink.

There are also more social media influencers and famous faces promoting wellness and health rather than drink and drugs. From Tyler, the Creator and Kendrick Lamar to Lana Del Rey and Blake Lively, celebrities are showing young people that you don't need alcohol to be successful. Like her or (more often than not) loathe her, Gwyneth and her Goop has also blazed a trail for like-minded wellness advocates to delve into retreats, crystals, holistic remedies, kale juices, organic products and expensive powders promising eternal youth. Likewise, influencers such as Ella Woodward (Deliciously Ella) and Brian Keane all promote healthy bodies and minds as the key to happiness. With so much positivity and education around health and wellness, it's hard to see how alcohol fits into the future like it has in the past.

Lisa Collins is the author of *The Man Who Moved the Nation: A Daughter's Story*, a book about losing her beloved father to cancer. As soon as her father had discovered that he had lung cancer brought about by smoking, he signed up to front a HSE campaign to create awareness of the dangers. Everyone who lived in Ireland in 2014 knew the ad and Lisa's dad. 'I wish I was an actor,' Gerry Collins began as he explained, face on to the camera, that he was dying as a result of cancer caused by smoking. Two months after

Gerry's ad first aired, he tragically lost his life. Gerry's legacy was to help over 100,000 people try to give up smoking.

When Lisa's book came out in 2018, I spoke to her about her continued link with the HSE, about smoking and about drinking. She had been chatting not long before to one of the managers in the HSE that the family had worked with on the campaign and alcohol had come up in the conversation.

'We're not ready,' the woman said. 'It has to be the right time for a campaign like that, and Ireland's not ready to look at its drinking habits just yet.'

I knew exactly what she meant.

But even in the short time since then, things have changed. In 2017, the Ask About Alcohol website was launched by the HSE. Their aim is to build awareness of the impact of alcohol on our health and wellbeing, and since then they have gone from strength to strength. Many in-depth surveys on our nation have shown that harmful drinking has become the norm for a large majority of us, yet many of the risks aren't widely known. We need to educate ourselves, build our knowledge, fill in the missing pieces.

'The HSE wants people to know about the direct connection between alcohol and cancer, alcohol and weight, alcohol and physical performance, alcohol and family life, and alcohol and mental health. It wants them to know more so that they can make informed choices about their own physical and mental health.'

Maybe we are finally ready.

The HSE isn't the only one who knows that changes are afoot. Sales of low- and non-alcoholic beer jumped by 60% in the Republic in 2018. In 2019, the Irish Brewers Association (IBA) forecast that more independent and craft producers were likely to follow in the footsteps of drinks giants such as Guinness in introducing low- and non-alcoholic beers. At the time of writing at the end of 2020, this has already happened with the likes of Irish craft breweries such Wicklow Wolf, Stonewell Cider and Brewmaster all bringing out their NA offerings.

On the global scale, just about every big brewer in the industry now has a version, including Heineken, Carlsberg, Budweiser, Stella Artois, Peroni, Cobra and Krombacher, to name just a few.

Why is this happening? Because there is money to be made. According to Fact.MR, global sales of low- and no-alcohol drinks are expected to surpass $28 billion by 2027. That is certainly worth jumping on the bandwagon for.

It will be interesting to see how the marketing of these offerings develops over time. Will it follow the same sexy, goodtime dreams of their alcohol-based counterparts? Advertising first began in America in the 1700s and billboards became the norm as early as the 1800s. The start of the 1900s saw brands like Kodak and Ford advertising their brand rather than just a product. In the 1920s, soap manufacturers began to sponsor weekly radio drama series, which then became known as 'soap operas'. The 1940s saw the first TV advert. And then psychologists got involved in the 1960s and everything changed. Focus groups, research, infomercials, massive marketing budgets and celebrity endorsements followed.

When we look back at some of those first ads from the past, we laugh. Cocaine toothache drops for kids promising an 'instantaneous cure', cola for babies for a 'better start in life', backed up, of course, by scientific research (from the Soda Pop Board of America, hmmm) that told us that it was 'proven that babies who start drinking soda during that early formative period have a much higher chance of fitting in and gaining acceptance during those awkward pre-teen and teenage years'. Cigarette brand Virginia Slims targeted the modern, independent woman with the tagline 'NEVER let the goody two shoes get you down'.

There are also plenty of deeply sexist, disturbing adverts like the one depicting a woman on the floor beside men's shoes being advertised: 'Keep her where she belongs...' Or another: 'You won him – now you must keep him.' Thanks, Lux. Or my personal favourite: 'A wife can blame herself if she loses love by getting "middle-age" skin.'

Thankfully, things have changed over the years. Advertising standards were brought in, meaning you couldn't make false claims around your product, so no more marketing smoking and cola as healthy or Guinness as being good for you. In the 1970s, print and TV ads for smoking were banned in the US. In recent years, even stricter laws have come in. In 2018, the Irish government passed the Public Health (Alcohol) Act, which prohibits alcohol advertising in or on public service vehicles, at public transport stops or stations, and within 200 metres of a school, crèche or local authority playground. Cinemas were stopped from advertising alcohol except around films with an age 18 classification. All children's clothing that promotes alcohol was prohibited.

Sounds obvious, doesn't it? But what about sporting events? Alcohol Action Ireland states:

> *Diageo, sponsor of Irish rugby and the Gaelic Athletic Association (GAA), attributes sales increases directly to sports sponsorship activity in its annual reporting and Carlsberg, sponsor of the FAI, in recent annual reports, have stated that 'ultimately, sponsorships are about growing our business and driving the long-term sales of our beer brands'.*

Advertising alcohol hand in hand with sports is an obvious contradiction. Will we look back on these advertisement deals in the same way as the outdated ads of the past and wonder incredulously, 'How was that allowed?!'

The same Public Health (Alcohol) Act also brought in minimum pricing and, controversially, a ruling regarding labelling on alcoholic drinks. Similar to warnings on cigarettes packaging, all alcohol products manufactured, imported or sold in the state will need to contain:

- A warning that is intended to inform the public of the danger of alcohol consumption
- A warning that is intended to inform of the dangers of alcohol consumption when pregnant
- The number of calories in the product and the number of grams in the product
- A link to a public health website, to be set up by the HSE, that will give information on alcohol- and other health-related harms.

It's all gentle steps in the direction of breaking the hold that alcohol has in our culture. It takes time, but as my friend Jill likes to say, 'It's directionally correct.'

There is one major global event, however, that could not have been predicted. That is, of course, the Covid-19 pandemic and the resulting lockdowns across countries and continents.

I recently listened to a podcast in which the non-drinking interviewee described it perfectly. When a friend asked him, 'How can you get through this without alcohol?', he replied, 'How can you get through this *with* alcohol?'

But we are in the minority. Alcohol use for many surged during the pandemic. The pub-shaped hole in people's lives was filled with at-home drinking instead. And with no morning rush to worry about during the first lockdown, everyone was struggling for an excuse *not* to reach for the bottle. No school run, no commute, no evening gym, no break from the monotony or the stress – no wonder so many people began to use a drink as the dividing line between working (from home) and not working (from home).

In the early months of the Covid-19 pandemic in Ireland, Drinkaware reported that one-quarter of Irish adults were drinking more than before. Frequency was one factor that contributed to this increase, with 14% drinking four or more times a week. The overwhelming reason that people were drinking was to help them unwind and relax. And with increased tensions in our homes and heads, God knows we all needed to do that.

In August, when the pubs debate was raging, Padraig Cribben, chief executive of the Vintners' Federation of Ireland, said that if alcohol was exacerbating the spread of Covid-19 and pubs were to be closed again, then restrictions of the sale of alcohol in off-licenses and supermarkets should be discussed. Basically it amounted to 'if we can't sell it, then nobody else should be able to either'. We didn't like that suggestion at all.

By the time the schools returned in August and September, parents around the country were rubbing their eyes and wondering whether it was time to get a handle on things and break those newly formed habits: Drinking during the week. Drinking more than before. Drinking to destress. Drinking to mark the end of the workday. Others waited for the 'back to the office, please!' email (which never came) to get a handle of things. Others, months later, are still struggling to. New routines have been formed. New stresses have emerged. Nerves are worn thin.

Then, as we approached the second lockdown in October, with all pubs and restaurants once again closing, the possibility of reducing the hours of off-licences was finally discussed. (The fact that they were designated 'essential' retailers was not.) We didn't like that suggestion either.

Like everything when it comes to our society's relationship with alcohol, it's complicated. Of those surveyed by Drinkaware in April 2020, 25% stated that their consumption had actually decreased and that they were taking this time to recalibrate. Even more than that felt that they had made positive changes to their drinking habits during lockdown. But during that month alone the Drinkaware website had almost 90,000 visits, proving that people were concerned about their drinking habits but were also proactively looking for ways to help themselves. We want it. We don't want it. We love it. We hate it.

The longer-term effects of lockdown and the pandemic still remain to be seen. Will it be a ripple or a tsunami? Will the increased reliance on alcohol lead to a spike in both physical and mental health issues? Will our country cope if it does?

It is interesting to think, though, how well equipped our health service would be to deal with this unprecedented phenomenon if alcohol-related illnesses weren't overrunning our society and our hospital beds.

Chapter 12

The Other Side

This morning I woke with the hazy September sunshine peeking in through the sides of the curtains. It's Sunday and the kids were all away last night, so the house is still. Aodhan and I drink coffee in bed and read the Sunday papers, luxuriating in the silence. When we've had our fill, we pull on some clothes and stroll down to the sea for our morning dip. The sun breaks through the clouds and the sea is a clear, deep blue, holding up handsome sailing boats. I take a deep breath and look to the distance, the horizon blending stripes of a perfectly curated palette. After, with salty skin and dripping hair, we walk back through the quiet streets and sit in the sunshine outside a café, drinking strong coffee and eating fruit scones, homemade jam dripping from my fingertips. I pop in to see my mother on the way home. 'Hold on,' she says, hurrying from the door. 'I'll just pause mass on my laptop.' A phrase I never thought I'd hear in my lifetime.

I go to collect the kids, tidy the kitchen, meal plan for the week, then sit down to write this. It's 3 p.m. and I have the rest of the day to still enjoy.

There's nothing remarkable in any of this, yet it ticks all the boxes that give me pleasure. Reading, connection, nature, exercise, food, family, home, writing.

I know they are only little things, but I feel an overwhelming sense of contentment and gratitude. The simple pleasures in life are never to be underestimated. Whether it's fresh clean sheets or fresh cut flowers, a sunrise or a sunset, perfecting the formation of a sentence in the written word or listening to the swell of a song you love, stroking the flushed cheek of a sleeping child or holding the well-worn hand of a loved one, the poetry of life is to be found in the power of small. And not drinking gives you so many more opportunities to find those moments.

Poetry is a beautiful thing, but you need time to really sit with the words, letting them permeate your body and soul in order to feel the full effect. The most perfectly crafted poem, when read in haste and agitation, loses all meaning and power. That's how I feel about life's simple pleasures. They need calm in order for you to be able to soak them up and appreciate them.

The bigger goals I've ticked off during my alcohol-free years – writing, running, swimming – all go back to my childhood loves. These were the things I knew I wanted to do when I was a young girl, before life got complicated. Before the grown-up pressures of careers, mortgages and children took hold. Before imposter syndrome, lethargy and time built up their imposing walls.

What did you love to do as a child? What did you want to achieve in life? Where did you picture yourself? Who did you want to become? There's something so simple but inherently authentic about returning to those childhood dreams. That's where we find our true selves. Perhaps you weren't sporty and writing wasn't your thing, but maybe you loved baking or you lost yourself in painting or music.

Most of us don't manage to make a career from our passions, and because of that we can lose them altogether. But the time, money and energy boosts that you get back from giving up alcohol could allow you to rekindle those loves again, which in turn make you feel more whole and your life more meaningful. Big claims that I promise are true.

* * *

Money isn't usually the main motivating factor in quitting the booze, but it's a very welcome side effect. Lots of people use it as a physical embodiment of the many benefits, a little like the apps that count up how many calories you have saved. So much of the good stuff relating to giving up drink is hard to quantify, so it's nice to have something tangible to reflect on. Calories and money are two factors that can be counted, whereas the internal and mental health benefits as well as energy, time and relationships can't be physically tracked so easily.

I have justified many a purchase over the years using my 'alcohol' fund, from getting a cleaner and starting a pension to booking regular massages. Fortunately, most of my chosen hobbies and goals are free – running, swimming and writing don't need much financial input – but using your savings to take guitar lessons or sign up to a course can meld the tangible gain (money) with the more empirical gains (time and energy) to create even more benefits (career progression, realisation of life goals, travel).

Or perhaps you just want to be able to buy yourself a new wardrobe or some new furniture. Being able to see a physical item that you were able to purchase as a side effect of not spending money on alcohol is a powerful talisman to carry with you.

Everyone will have their own list of life improvements that they want to tackle in their alcohol-free travels. It could be anything from not hating yourself anymore to starting your own business. There's no right or wrong, just your own desires.

But don't just take my word for it. I've gathered stories from four others who have chosen to take the road less travelled too.

Jennifer

If you had told me a few years ago that I'd be a non-drinker in the future, I would have probably spat out my wine from laughing so hard! Yet here I am, almost four years without any alcohol, and I'm loving life in the biggest, brightest, shout-it-from-the-rooftops way!

There was no big event that caused me to want to take this break. No rock bottom, no hangovers or crumbling life. I have a happy marriage, a wonderful kid and a productive, active life. But I felt like something was holding me back from being the best version of myself. I felt like alcohol was becoming too much of who I was. Too much of what defined me or what people identified me with – someone who likes her wine. It seemed like an uninspiring, boring, unimaginative hobby, not to mention unhealthy. I started to question my drinking habits when I found myself looking forward a little too much to my evening glasses of wine, or planning an extra trip to the store to grab a bottle, or thinking that it helped to deal with life's speed bumps in any way, shape or form. It felt like maybe I was depending on it a little too much and I did not like the idea of something having control over me. Plus I had young eyes watching and learning from me, and drinking was also keeping me from reaching health and fitness goals. Stress, celebrations, watching sunsets, getting good news (or bad news), vacations, going out to dinner, hanging out with friends – these were all occasions in my mind to justify a few drinks, and those drinks add up fast over the course of a week.

I was of the mindset that alcohol soothed the bad times, enhanced the good times and helped me to relax in the evenings. I quickly learned that I couldn't have been more wrong.

Deciding to ditch alcohol was a catalyst for so much growth and discovery and I learned to love myself in a way I never had before. It pushed me to challenge myself in other areas and to use what I've learned to accomplish other big goals, like running a marathon, going vegetarian and getting in shape. Little did I know that I was practising for the biggest test of my life, watching my dad lose his battle with cancer. I'm forever grateful that I wasn't still under the impression that alcohol made things easier. Because I had learned so much about myself, I was able to be the best healthcare advocate for him, be there by his side for the six months of his battle, hold his hand while he took his last breath and not think of drinking once! I was able to grieve in the healthiest way possible and be there for my mom. That is so huge to me.

The biggest, most profound transformation from quitting drinking, for me, came from within. When you feel so good on the inside, you can't help but look in the mirror and feel proud and at peace with the reflection that is staring back at you, through the good times and bad and everything in between. I know I am strong and capable of getting through anything!

These days, my buzz is natural and long lasting. My laughter comes from an authentic place. I learned to love and accept myself more. I learned to make time for myself, to fuel my body better and to deal with setbacks and stressors in a healthy way.

And last but not least, I learned that it was never, ever the wine that made the occasion more fun. It was the company I kept, the meaningful friendships, the conversations and laughter, the activities I was doing and the occasions I was celebrating. It was never the wine that soothed the heartache and tears. It was being true to my emotions and not numbing a damn moment. It was learning to say 'what is this moment trying to teach me?' rather than 'why is this happening to me?'. Taking a break from alcohol is a gift I gave myself that I get to unwrap and enjoy each and every day!

Jo

I was actually relatively late to the whole drinking scene – about 16 years old. Although it sounds crazy to me now, most of my friends would have started much earlier than that. From that moment on there was no stopping me, though. I drank at parties, in fields, on weekends, in pubs, at happy hour and lunch dates throughout my teens, twenties and thirties. I appeared to be the life and soul at every occasion (unless I was asleep …) and didn't stop to question it. But as the years went on, the secret I was keeping from those around me got louder and louder.

I didn't actually like myself very much, and alcohol made it worse.

I was tired of feeling anxious, wracked with self-loathing every weekend and terrified of who I would meet when I went to Tesco to do the family shop. What if I had said something offensive or had done something stupid the night or week before, or sometime in the past I couldn't remember? Blackouts were a regular thing and I thought everyone had them.

When I gave up drinking, it was hard at first. People would offer me pints in the pub and coax me into having 'just one'. They told me they missed the old me and asked when she would be coming back. She was much more fun. No one wanted the non-drinker in their midst. I knew this feeling well, as I'd done the same to my friend who'd given up before me. Once, at a friend's wedding, I was seated beside a guy I had never met before. We hit it off, chatting and laughing for the whole meal – until someone mentioned that I didn't drink. 'You don't drink?' he said incredulously before instantly moving away and clearly avoiding me for the remainder of the evening. I didn't think I was less fun, it was simply other people's perceptions of me. It was their problem, not mine.

But it wasn't easy.

A few months after giving up, it was New Year's Eve and stupidly I thought I would just do what I always did – celebrate it with friends. Despite the fact that I have never enjoyed New Year's Eve and would have preferred to be at home in my pyjamas with a takeaway.

A large group of us gathered in the local pub and within a couple of hours I knew I was not comfortable, so I went out for a walk. I walked the streets for an hour, taking big gulps of cold air and quietly crying. I think I was grieving the past and my place in it. Finding out who you are without alcohol is a massive journey and it takes time, patience and acceptance. There's also no hiding from the hard stuff. Grief, pain, worry – they all need to be felt and processed. When I lost my beloved mother, the force of the feelings shocked me, but I was also full of gratitude that I was fully there with her – and that I honoured her loss with the pain I felt, fully and deeply.

I'm now four years alcohol free and have no intention or desire ever to drink again. I actually like myself now, which is a massive thing for me to be able to say. I spent far too long feeling the opposite way. What an absolute waste.

I can honestly say that I am happier in myself and I know myself at a much deeper level now – and sure, isn't that what life is all about? It took 25 years for me to realise drink didn't suit me, but I had fun acting like a Rolling Stone until I got there!

Lisa

I've always associated having a good time with drinking. Not a daily drinker (or even weekly necessarily), but I almost always overdid it once I decided to have a night out or a few drinks.

I did about six weeks alcohol free during lockdown and really enjoyed it but I had no real plan. I went for a walk with a friend and we stopped to sit and admire the view and he took out a bottle of beer for each for us. I accepted it without even thinking and that was the end of the non-drinking for the next two months. I had just taken it out of his hand and drank it without even noticing – how conditioned is that?!

I also increasingly noticed myself not having a good

time where alcohol was involved. Two or three times over the summer, I distinctly noticed that I was really uncomfortable being around it.

I have a good job, am well respected in work circles and well paid, own a nice house – these things have happened almost in spite of myself. I am a bit overwhelmed by what is possible with a clear head – on a personal level but also in society as a whole. This is going to take me time to work through.

I now know (and probably always did) what is possible for me. I don't think I can go back to accepting less for myself – relationships (romantic or otherwise), work, believing harsh comments, drifting along, etc. By raising the bar, my daughter's whole life and expectations will be raised without her even being aware. I also need to process that – it's pretty huge, but kind of makes my heart thump faster too. Is this 'doing the work'?

I don't think it's as simple as saying that removing alcohol has given me all the benefits I'll list, but removing it has made me focus more on my life and being happy, which in turn has brought these changes:

Walked well over 300,000 steps – barely remember any of them; it really is one step at a time!

Lost 8 pounds.

Lots of sea swimming and walking on the beach and in the forest.

Cooked all our meals.

Have been a better mum and better friend (mostly to myself).

Have begun removing myself from a friendship that has been dragging me down.

Have had dozens of moments of wondering 'is this real life?'.

Caught myself saying out loud to the dog on the way down the stairs, 'Right. Let's set our intentions for the day!'

Completed work projects with ease – find myself wondering what it was that I found difficult about my job.

Almost by chance earned nearly €1,000 from a sideline piece of work, something that flew out of me so well that I'm considering if I should look into creating an actual side business.

Since the first week, I have been fully awake as soon as I wake up and am usually out of bed by 6 a.m.

Life is good.

Maeve

Like most Irish people, I grew up surrounded by alcohol. When I was a child, my father used to brew his own wine and I remember the huge brown jars, which he would attend to with care, fermenting in the hot press. I imagine the home brewing had a lot to do with the cost of wine in 1980s Ireland. I was given my first drink – a West Coast Cooler – by an older friend when I was 13. I distinctly remember the giddy feeling, the rush of warmth, and feeling like a grown-up. As the fourth child in a family of five, being treated as grown-up, or feeling like one, wasn't something I was used to and I liked it.

I didn't drink a lot in secondary school, but I made up for it when I went to college. Drinking to excess seemed to be normal, or rather, it was normalised. There were 'pound a drink' nights in pubs and nightclubs, and drinking doubles made more sense than queueing at the bar for ages. Most nights out were a blur – reconstructing and deconstructing the previous night was part of the craic. I graduated, but I certainly didn't do myself justice with my results.

Once I started working, socialising always revolved around alcohol. Nights at the pub midweek, then on the weekends, we would drink at home while getting ready, then head into the pub, followed by a nightclub, then more drinks at home. Every single weekend night out was binge drinking, according to the guidelines (more than three alcoholic drinks at one time), but since everyone else was doing it, that made it okay, right?

Once I had kids my consumption dropped, at least for a time. I didn't drink while I was pregnant or breastfeeding, but apart from that, alcohol continued to play too large a part in my life. I had taken up running, which I felt was almost a justification for continuing to drink. I was slim and exercising regularly, so I must have been healthy! I would joke about preferring to drink my calories, but it wasn't a joke. I would reduce the calories I got from food (actual nutrition!) so that I could drink the empty calories in wine. My husband (who is also a runner) and I would joke about running to sweat out the red wine so that we could make room for more.

Meeting the girls meant wine. A stressful day at work meant wine. Dinner out with my husband meant wine. A midweek movie on the couch meant wine. Kids acting out and driving me crazy meant wine. It seemed impossible to consider that any of these activities could be enjoyed, or any of these incidents endured, without wine. That's largely because of the bullshit tropes we are sold through advertising and popular culture about how wine relaxes us, makes life more effervescent and enjoyable, makes parenting kids bearable. It's all untrue, and it's revolting.

The truth was, my tolerance was increasing, I was drinking wine four or five nights out of seven and I felt like shit. I wasn't sleeping properly. I had low-grade anxiety most of the time and worst of all, I was sleepwalking through the day to get to five o'clock, when it became socially acceptable to have a drink. (Apart from brunch on the weekends, when apparently it's okay to drink wine in the morning as long as it's mixed with juice. This is not okay, people! It's socially acceptable, but it's not okay.) I was irritable with my kids and my sense of self was slowly eroding. I was starting to let people in my personal life treat me badly because I felt so guilty and shameful about my drinking. My thinking was: I was a drinker, I was reliant on a substance, therefore I must also be at fault in all other situations. I had a problem.

There was no rock bottom for me (thank God). I am a well-paid, highly respected professional and a valued member of my team. I have never lost a job or been reprimanded for any performance issue at any time because of my drinking. I have a happy, successful marriage and three smart, kind, healthy, active kids. So I don't fit the typical image of an alcoholic, and now that I have done a LOT of reading around alcohol, I know that I'm not one. Alcohol is a highly addictive, socially endorsed, carcinogenic neurotoxin that is marketed to us (particularly women) by an insidious multibillion-dollar drinks industry. I am not the problem. Alcohol is the problem.

There are a couple of key moments that made me decide I needed to stop drinking. Visiting family and friends on a longed-for two-week trip one summer resulted in too many heavy nights out and me in tears on one of those nights after a minor disagreement with my eldest sister. Over what? I have no idea. I stopped drinking after that for a few months, but started drinking again as the Christmas party season ramped up as I had no alcohol-free support network and I didn't have any of the information that I would need to stay sober.

Then in May of this year a dear friendship ruptured, most spectacularly. The loss of this person from my life triggered an intense emotional response in me, mainly because of a previous loss that is still too painful for me to talk about in a public forum. I was a mess, filled with grief and pain. So I drank. But I realised that this poison was not making me feel better – it was in fact making me feel much, much, much worse. It wasn't helping me to cope, it was making it harder to cope. All the emotions were still there the following day, only magnified, and I was even less able to deal with them. I had been avoiding the One Year No Beer ads of my Facebook feed for many months, but one Saturday morning, 22 May 2020, I joined up and I haven't touched a drop of alcohol since.

The biggest challenge I've faced is managing my emotions. I think a lot of people drink because we lack the other tools we need to deal with difficult emotions like anger, resentment or grief. We're not taught this stuff anywhere, rarely in our family of origin, certainly not in school! We don't have the skills to name what we're feeling and to process in a healthy way what we are going through. I used to scoff at people who meditated or did yoga or read self-help books or journaled, but guess what? That shit works far better than alcohol and it doesn't kill you, so that's nice. I'm a work in progress for sure. I'm still developing self-differentiation (basically how not to get consumed by other people's emotions) and self-regulation (how not to turn to external sources for soothing when stressed), but every day I'm more centred, more certain of myself.

Alcohol-free life is better in absolutely every way and that's not an exaggeration. Relationships are better. I'm calmer and I'm a more focused and present parent. I still want to kill the husband from time to time, but sure, that's normal. I'm more present to him too and more likely to suggest date nights or new, fun activities. I'm more engaged and productive at work. I feel more confident in my judgement and my abilities. I have more energy. I sleep better. I'm just as funny when socialising and I remember every detail of the night. Crucially, I get to leave when nights out stop being fun. Orgasms are easier to attain and are more intense. I am able to stick to exercise schedules without dread, and if I do miss a session, I don't beat myself up about it. There is no shame and guilt spiral. If I make a mistake, at least I know it's not due to being hungover, so I can learn from it in a meaningful way. My friends don't care that I don't drink, although I know that's not everyone's experience. I haven't had to develop other friendships because there was, and is, real value in those I have; it was never just about the booze. I enjoy food now – like, I *really* enjoy it. It tastes better and is relished and remembered rather than just being soakage or extra calories I worried about consuming.

I know I sound like a zealot, and of course there is still grief and pain as well as the irritations and frustrations that regularly come with being a human. But now I feel better able to cope with them. Ultimately, all I can say is that I'm finally living an authentic life that's actually based on my values and desires, not on automatic responses or the need for a drink. And I'm happy.

* * *

I recognise parts of myself in all these stories. For many of us there was no rock bottom, no stereotypical red flags that we associate with alcoholism, no major drama. There was just a low hum of discontent in the background of our busy lives. For the majority of Irish and British people, our drinking habits aren't so bad that we are forced to stop. On the contrary, our drinking habits are regular and normalised, so why *would* we stop?

But there is a definite shift in the atmosphere. Changes are afoot. More and more people are questioning their relationship with alcohol.

So where do you start if you're sober curious?

What this whole experience has taught me is that it's not just a certain type of person that can quit drinking. I never, ever thought I would be a non-drinker, yet here I am. And so many others who chose to stop feel exactly the same way. We were just like you. So whether you are an everyday drinker, a weekend lush, a party binger, a red wine snob or a gin aficionado, you can still do it. It can be very daunting starting out, though, so here are some tips to keep you from stumbling off the path in the early days.

Nights Out

It can be a good idea to avoid nights out at the start, though not for too long. Learning to socialise without alcohol is important – you can't hide away forever! Why not get one or two weekends under your belt before tackling the pub or restaurant social scene? That's not to say you have to become a hermit in that time – you can always see if friends are free to go for a hike or grab a coffee instead. Post-Covid this has become the norm anyway, so use this opportunity to normalise it.

Once you decide to embark on a night out, choose it carefully. Make sure it's with people you feel comfortable spending time with. It might sound a bit over the top, but having a pre-prepared script in your head can also be useful. Have an answer ready for the inevitable 'How come you're not drinking?' question. Know what drink you are going to order and have a back-up in case they don't stock it. Most pubs and restaurants now have a selection of alcohol-free options available. In the past I've even run next door to the local off-licence to bring my own AF beers into a restaurant that didn't have any on the menu. They were very apologetic and popped the bottles in the fridge for me. On my next visit they had added AF choices to the list. Ireland is changing, but some establishments may still need a friendly reminder.

Have an exit strategy planned. By midnight you will likely be exhausted and conversations will begin to get messy. Will you slip out unnoticed or give a firm 'I'm off' as you pull on your coat? A word of warning: offering lifts can be a minefield. No one will be ready to go when you are and you'll likely end up stressed and resentful while you wait for them to 'just finish this drink'. They, on the other hand, will find you annoying and boring for making them leave before they are ready.

I usually whisper to one trusted person that I'm off and then no one even notices that you're gone. The good old Irish Goodbye lives on.

The Spanish Inquisition

Sometimes it's on a night out, but it can happen at any time: the barrage of questions that say more about the person asking than the fact that you're not drinking.

'What do you mean you're not drinking?' 'Why aren't you drinking? You're not an alcoholic.' 'Is this a health thing?' 'Did something happen?' 'Are you pregnant?' 'Can we still be friends?' 'How long is this for?' 'Will you not just have one?'

As a culture, we can be very defensive about our drinking habits. If you change yours, it holds a mirror up to those around you, and most often they don't like it. You've shaken up the status quo and made them ask themselves questions they don't want to have to answer. Having ready responses that don't judge, blame or preach can help. If you are clear and confident in your answering, it's much less likely that they will persist. I remember when my kids were all young being advised by a more experienced mother to never show any hesitation if answering 'no' to a child's request – they can smell the indecision and will go in for the kill, pestering until they get their way. It's a little like that. Be firm and don't show any sign of weakness and everyone will move on to other matters.

Boredom

One of the main reasons people don't fulfil their resolution to give up drink is because of the perceived boredom. We spend a significant amount of our time drinking, so when we get back all that time, we need something to fill the void. Having a project or a goal – whether it's fitness, creative or career focused – will make a big difference in how your challenge goes.

Most of us can drop the drink from our weekday schedules easily enough, but the weekends are a whole other story. Pre-empt the boredom with plans. A gallery visit, a long walk, a football match, a shopping trip, visiting friends – have something fun planned to mark your day with. Evenings can be filled with the cinema, a takeaway or a home spa until you're ready to face more social occasions.

If you normally drink at home on Friday and Saturday nights, make sure you buy in some alcohol-free options. Test out a few every week and find your favourites. It's surprising how a Seedlip and tonic in a cut glass tumbler can feel just as good as the real thing or how easily a bottle of Open Gate Pure Brew can replace your usual beer choice.

Stress

Identifying your triggers and finding substitutes for dealing with them also helps in those early weeks. If you normally reach for the bottle after a bad day, you will need to find other ways of dealing with the stress. A walk, a run, a swim, a phone call, a bath, scented candles, crystals, cleaning, meditation, going for a drive, listening to music – there are lots of options. You just might need to retrain your brain in order to find them.

My current favourites are a freezing swim in the morning that takes me from bad mood bear to ready to take on the world. At lunchtime I put my headphones in and take a looped walk around the seafront of my town. In the evenings I put some drops of bergamot, grapefruit or lavender essential oil in my diffuser, light some candles and have a bath. I will often have an alcohol-free beer and some posh crisps in the evening, but it would no longer cross my mind to have an alcoholic beer. The need for that release is no longer there because I get the release in other ways now. It's all about forming new habits.

Partners

I was really lucky in that I took this trip with Aodhan. I've no doubt at all that it would be tougher doing it alone. I've heard stories of supportive partners and of those that were deeply offended. If you're in a relationship with someone who drinks, then there's a good chance that much of your bonding is done around it. It's not just our own identities that are immersed in alcohol – our relationships are too.

If you have a partner who is against your decision, it makes for a much tougher journey. To combat this, try to really dig down into the reasons why you want to do this and then explain it to them. Perhaps write it all down and ask them to read it. Ask them to think about why they don't want you to do this – is it because they fear that it will impact your relationship? That they don't want you to see them drunk when you are sober? That you won't be able to bond like before? Talk it out – make them ask those questions of themselves. It may lead to fascinating insights. Ask them to join a sober Facebook group, read up on sober curious articles or listen to alcohol-free discussions and podcasts. This may be the first time in your entire lives that you have questioned alcohol, so give them time to catch up with where you are.

*   *   *

Scattered. That's the word that best described me in the past. Whether this manifested itself externally, I'm not sure, but internally that's how I felt. My mood and mind were constantly jumping from one thing to another.

I now feel calm.

I still have bad days. I still feel all the emotions. We're not supposed to be happy all the time. Life is fear, and sadness, and excitement, and guilt. Emotions are there to be felt and experienced – that *is* life. We don't default to happy and we're not broken or failing if we feel other things instead of it.

I'm now grateful for my calm. For my quietness. It's who I really am. I spent too many years trying to force myself into a more vivacious shape – and why? Because society places more values on extroverts? Most of the people I have met or heard stories from in the non-drinking community were all doing the same thing too – trying to be more *something*. More something that they weren't. Now they have accepted who they are and lean into that.

I like books and poetry and nature and peace. It was true of me when I was a child and it's still true of me now. Did I lose sight of my true self because of alcohol? Did I begin to drift away from myself as a teenager, trying to fit into a box that wasn't made for me? Those boxes that we often find ourselves in are so small, so restricting, that we wake up one day and wonder who the hell we are and how the hell we got here. And then, mostly subconsciously, we use alcohol to numb that feeling. It's often the knowledge that something isn't right. An itch that we don't want to scratch because the answer might turn out to be just too scary. When we are teens alcohol helps us to be someone we are not by giving us false confidence, until slowly we lose sight of who we truly are. And then we simply don't know how to go back.

I started to drink because everyone else was doing it. And they started because everyone before them was doing it. And on and on back through the generations. It reminds me of the five monkeys experiment.

A researcher puts five monkeys in a cage. He hangs a bunch of bananas above a stepladder in the cage. When the first monkey begins to climb the ladder to get to the bananas, the researcher sprays all the monkeys with freezing cold water. A little later, another monkey decides he'll have a go and begins to climb the ladder. Again, all five monkeys are sprayed with freezing water. But when the next monkey decides that he will try to get the bananas, a funny thing happens. The researcher does not have to spray them at all – the other monkeys stop him themselves. They are afraid that they will get sprayed again, so they pull him back down. The five monkeys have learned not to climb the ladder.

Next, the researcher replaces one of the original monkeys with a new monkey. This monkey has never experienced the freezing water spray, so obviously he goes to climb the ladder to get the bananas. As soon as he does, the other monkeys attack – they all remember the freezing water and don't want to get sprayed again. And so the new monkey learns not to try to climb the ladder either.

The researcher then replaces another of the original monkeys with a new monkey. He, too, tries to get to the bananas and he, too, is attacked by the other monkeys – *including* the new monkey who was never sprayed with water.

One by one, each of the original monkeys is replaced with a new monkey until none of the original five remain. Each time the newest member in the cage goes for the bananas, they are attacked despite none of the monkeys in the cage ever having experienced the cold water spray.

Why do they attack? Because they've all learned from their peers that *that's the way it's done around here.*

And so they all remain grounded, unable to reach for that which will sustain them and make them feel good. Scared to climb the ladder to get a better view.

That's all of us. Following the crowd because that's the way it's done, continually dragging each other back to the status quo, oblivious to the fact that there is another way – one with a better view and far nicer rewards.

✳ ✳ ✳

Last night I came home from the boys' football run to find Aodhan lying on the bed doing Wim Hof deep breathing and listening to a Tibetan bowls and gongs playlist on Spotify. Instead of laughing at him or running from the room in horror, I lay down on the bed beside him, placed one of his earphones into my ear and joined in. In the darkness I filled my belly and chest with a deep breath, let the reverberations of the powerful sounds course through my body and felt the huge grin spread across my face.

Not your usual Thursday evening, that's for sure, but we get our kicks where we can these days. We've both discovered and delved into more interests in the past four years than ever before and learned so much about ourselves and our world along the way.

When I stop to take stock of my life, which I do often these days, I am so grateful for this second chance, this unexpected freedom that I have been gifted, this accidentally sober path I stumbled on. I didn't even know that I was chained up until I escaped.

It doesn't feel like I am missing out or that I am living a good life *in spite of* not drinking. My life is infinitely better in every respect *because of* not drinking. I *choose* this. I choose early morning sunrises. I choose energy and productivity. I choose fitness and feeling good. I choose real friendships and deeper relationships. I choose music and food and art. I choose poetry and nature. I choose health and happiness and self-discovery.

What will you choose?

Acknowledgements

First, a huge thanks to Nicki Howard at Gill Books for trusting that I could write this book, even when I wasn't sure myself. I was truly humbled by the amount of thought, effort and professionalism by the whole team at Gill Books, especially Sarah Liddy (the only one I got to actually meet in person in between lockdowns!), Catherine Gough for her incredible and always spot-on editing skills and advice, Bartek Janczak for the internal design and Anna Morrison for the beautiful cover, and Avril Cannon for her fabulous marketing and PR prowess (I'll see you on the beach one of these days, Avril).

Thanks to my partner, Aodhan, for taking the trip with me – I don't think I would have lasted even a month without you – and for always supporting my writing efforts, even when your belief is not fully deserved.

Kristian and Liam, you both made the idea of not drinking an actual possibility – trailblazers.

My sisters, Siobhan and Maria – I knew you'd come around in the end.

To my friends who didn't desert me, and to those who let me write about them – thank you.

And sorry, Mum, for uncovering those childhood memories and putting them into print.

Thanks to One Year No Beer for helping me along at the start, especially Andy Ramage, and Community Manager Barbara Fitzsimons for sending me so many positive stories to choose from for the final chapter. Your members are truly inspirational.

Finally, thanks to my kids for putting up with their embarrassing mum (and sorry you've no drinks cabinet to raid during your teenage years).